TESTIMONIALS

Testimony from clients and students who have
experienced and applied Garcia Innergetics

Garcia Innergetics went beyond any expectations I had. The acceleration achieved within the Innergetic morphic field is very obvious and sacred. I see the difference; the knowingness and energies that work to honor what you are all become available through this method. Dr. Garcia facilitates our ability to change the universe and ourselves. His work is a huge blessing to us all, and his respect and responsibility for that work and the tools he shares is awesome and unique. Thank you.

—Joe

Garcia Innergetics is informative and easy to follow. I can implement the tools Dr. Garcia shares to better my life. I am thrilled.

—Anne

Dr. Garcia offers great attention to detail. The personal corrections and healings I've received have been very good. Garcia Innergetics is one of the best experiences I've had with this work in twenty-nine years.

—Paul

I had a health issue that was corrected through Garcia Innergetics, and felt awesome after applying this work. I've learned how to harmonize, correct, and transform other people's issues, as well. Dr. Garcia's teachings are easy and simple to use in my everyday life.

—Gene

Garcia Innergetics and learning about my true "GPS" satisfy what my spirit has been wanting me to get, and to know.

—*Lisa*

I wasn't sure what to expect from Garcia Innergetics. Nevertheless, in a sense it has exceeded my expectations in that I've learned new tools that I didn't realize I needed. Thanks to Dr. Garcia I have recognized my blocks to doing this work, and I've gained so many insights! Thank you.

—*Melody*

Garcia Innergetics opened my world; what more could I want?! It's all starting to happen. I will be able to incorporate Dr. Garcia's knowledge on how to work with energy and his way of testing energy with my Reiki clients.

—*Lynn*

The wealth of information Dr. Garcia has tapped into with Garcia Innergetics is very powerful. It allows the energetic field to help us to access it. Dr. Garcia's method has a truth about it, and it's fun to "test" energy with these tools. Thank you.

—*Anonymous*

I once suffered from a very poor quality of life. I had been quite ill with hepatitis C for a number of years. I was also in constant pain as the result of an accident. Traditional western medicine had not helped much. I knew in my heart that somewhere there was someone with the knowledge and skill to help me, but I didn't know where to look. Then I found Dr. Garcia. Dr. Garcia recognizes that people are multifaceted beings; we are much more than physical bodies. His method, Garcia Innergetics, addresses the entire person—mental, spiritual, and physical—to provide care that is far superior to allopathic treatment alone. Now when my gastroenterologist, who doesn't believe in holistic medicine, says that I should have been dead years ago, I just smile. I know why I'm still alive. I'm here thanks to Dr. Garcia's God-given gifts.

—*M.M.*

As a former athlete suffering from premature career-ending injuries, I am extremely grateful to Dr. Garcia. Through an extremely effective blend of oriental medicine, unrivaled intuition, and innovative techniques, he has allowed me to recover from what seemed chronic, life-lasting issues. Garcia Innergetics has had a profound positive impact not only on my health, but also on my well-being and that of my family, across all walks of life.

—*Robert*

As an executive at a Fortune 100 company, the ability to make day-to-day decisions with confidence is critical. Since meeting Dr. Garcia and taking part in Garcia Innergetics, I have been able to learn how to harmonize energy to bring about fair outcomes and turn even the biggest adversity into an opportunity. I can't praise Dr. Garcia's work enough and I encourage everyone who wants to make a difference in this world to become familiar with his method, as it is truly a life-changer.

—*Alan*

I went to Dr. Garcia after facing a breast cancer diagnosis. I am deeply grateful for everything he did for me and still does. He is not just a "body-healer"; he makes no separation between soul, spirit, and body. His passion, mission, and will is to help his patients. He taught me that how I react to situations makes all the difference. I can't thank him enough for taking such good care of me.

—*Chichi*

I would like to express my immense gratitude to Dr. Garcia for his amazing talents and the gifts of his teachings through

Garcia Innergetics. I have had several profound and personal experiences as a result of Dr. Garcia's work in my life. His method has also empowered me to help others as a healer. One client of mine experienced a fall while she was snowboarding that dislocated her left shoulder, as seen on X-ray. I applied Dr. Garcia's method, and a few days later she returned to see me, saying that her orthopedic specialist had told her that the dislocated shoulder no longer existed. I was astonished that the energy was able to change so quickly and completely.

—Adam

I've been a neuromuscular therapist for twenty-one years and have always had recurring clients who re-injure the same areas. I was never able to figure out their issues completely. Since studying Garcia Innergetics, I have completely shifted and taken my clients to the next level in their recovery and healing on all levels—mentally, physically, and spiritually.

—Anonymous

Garcia Innergetics has completely shifted my life and business on a cellular level. Thank you Dr. Garcia.

—Amanda

I have been a student and patient of Dr. Garcia's for several years. During that time, I have gone through very profound shifts in my life. I have experienced a feeling of coming home to my Self and a greater sense of my connection with all. The work I have done with Garcia Innergetics has greatly facilitated this process, and I am very grateful to Dr. Garcia for all the guidance and support I've received during this time.

—J.D.

GUIDING
PERSONAL SOURCE

An Intuitive Healing Path to
Clarity, Balance, and Empowerment

DR. HECTOR E. GARCIA, D.C.

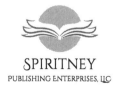

SPIRITNEY
PUBLISHING ENTERPRISES, LLC

San Diego, California

Spiritney Publishing Enterprises, LLC
P.O. Box 722286
San Diego, CA 92172
Phone +1 (858)450-9221

Limit of Liability/Disclaimer of Warranty:
The material contained in this book is intended to be educational and not for diagnosis, prescription or treatment of any health condition or disorder. This information should not replace the consultation with a licensed healthcare professional. The intent of the author is only to offer information of a general nature to help you in your quest for health, emotional and spiritual well being. The use of any of the information or other contents of this book, the author and the publisher assume no responsibility or liability.

Publishing and editorial team: Author Bridge Media,
                    www.AuthorBridgeMedia.com
Project Manager and Editorial Director: Helen Chang
Editor: Kristine Serio
Publishing Manager: Laurie Aranda
Publishing Assistant: Iris Sasing
Design: Six Penny Graphics

Library of Congress Control Number: 2016904052
ISBN: 978-0-9972659-0-3   -- softcover
         978-0-9972659-1-0   -- hardcover
         978-0-9972659-2-7   -- ebook
1. Holistic. 2. Energy Healing. 3. Self-help Personal. 4. Transformational.
5. Healing. 6. Consciousness. 7. Chakras

I dedicate this book to the spirit of my daughter, Hannah, and to my wife, Yolanda. Thank you for all that you do for me. Your love, support, and patience made this book possible.

Acknowledgments

This book would not have happened without the support and encouragement of many people in my life.

To my wife Yolanda for supporting me throughout the creation of this book, I am especially grateful.

I would also like to thank the following individuals, who played a role in helping me develop *Guiding Personal Source*, challenging me to tell my story.

Thank you to my nephews, Michael and Alex, for all your technical support and help. To my good friend and colleague Dr. John Hernandez, I thank you for our memorable conversations. I am grateful to Jennifer Joe for her networking expertise and connections, to Elsa and Mike Horvath for their commitment and support in this journey, and to Gerry and Joyce Tracey for their support and friendship. I am also grateful to all my clients, students, and mentors. And finally, thank you to Helen Chang, Kristine Serio, and the Author Bridge Media team for your editorial and publishing services.

CONTENTS

INTRODUCTION

Miracles within You

Miracles exist within you.

These miracles flow from an **energetic field** to which you are connected. Using this field, you have the ability to identify, improve, and even transcend any health issue in an instant. With it, ailments that used to be considered insurmountable are now no more difficult to address than a common cold. This energetic field is designed specifically for you, and you have access to it any time, day or night. You can access it wherever you are, and using it is easier than taking a deep breath and letting it go.

All of this is already yours: part and parcel of your intuition. Through it, you have access to the single most powerful energetic force that humankind has ever had, or ever will have. You were born with it. You've been carrying it with you all these years, maybe never even realizing that you were sitting on a goldmine.

Instead, you may have been searching for solutions to your health issue outside yourself. You may have seen doctors, specialists, naturopaths, and alternative health practitioners. Some of them may have helped you and some may not have. A few may have even told you point blank, "This is a condition you will have to deal with for the rest of your life."

Perhaps even the people who have helped you haven't really fixed the root of the problem. They've eased the symptoms, but the issue is still there. You may feel a little better, but you aren't *actually* better—yet.

You've been searching for a miracle, and that miracle does exist. However, you won't find it in anyone else's hands. The transformation you're looking for is within you, and it has been all along.

All you need to do is learn how to access it.

An Energetic Path to Healing

Everything is energy. That includes you, and it also includes your health condition. When you learn how to work with the energy fields that you are already in and part of, you empower yourself to build a personalized, energetic path to healing.

How can that be?

We think of health as physical, and we do manifest physical symptoms. But we are more than just our physical bodies. Our bodies are connected to our minds, and beyond that, to our spirits. The spiritual part of you is infinite, and it has access to infinite knowledge—including the answers you're seeking for your health.

The same health issue can be caused by any number of different things, both on and off the body. As I share in chapter 6, medical research is a useful resource, but it only scratches the surface of what's really going on with your health, because it's limited to physical observation.

By contrast, your personal energetic makeup can tell you exactly where the problem is coming from in your specific case. Moreover, it can harmonize the energy so that the issue no longer exists. In other words, when you approach your health with this method, you are not just covering up your symptoms. You are hitting an energetic reset button that actually causes them to diminish or disappear altogether, much like you'd hit the reset button on a computer program.

In other words, you no longer just *feel* better. You *are* better.

And that's only the beginning of how working with energy can transform your life.

Energy Facilitator

I've been a facilitator of energy my whole life—literally.

I was born intuitive, and as a child I was able to sense energy fields and harmonize them to help my friends, my family, and myself. As I grew up, I began to gear my abilities toward the healing sciences. I studied all the regular subjects—biochemistry, biology, physical therapy—but even though they had their merits, they were also limiting. They never ventured beyond what you could physically see, and I knew that much more than that was available.

So I set out to take the science of medicine to the next level by tapping into those other areas of energetic information.

Today, I've been in practice for more than twenty-five years. During that time, I've worked with thousands of people one on one, and countless others have been touched by my work through classes, workshops, teleconference calls, and other channels. I've facilitated the healing of everything from common colds to terminal conditions, as well as life issues that reach beyond the sphere of health alone.

In 2010, I launched *Garcia Innergetics* as a way to teach my evolving modality of energy work to others. Thousands of people have been through my courses, learned my method of facilitating energy, and taken that knowledge out into the world with inspiring results.

In my practice, I never assume anything about the symptoms people come in with. Assumptions are limiting. Instead, I allow the clients' energy to tell me why their symptoms are showing up, and why those symptoms are important in the bigger picture of people's lives. From there, I'm able to harmonize their energetic fields with effortless ease, and they can feel the results immediately.

You have the ability to do exactly the same thing.

Let Your Consciousness Be Your Guide

This book is not designed to teach you a step-by-step, one-size-fits-all system for working with energy. Instead, it will ignite the knowledge that already exists in you, so that you can guide yourself back to your original perfected essence, which includes a state of strong health and well-being. Even though the words may look the same for everyone on the surface, you will receive them in a way that specifically fits you.

You can **test** this for yourself, here and now.

Pause for a moment and think of something that is important to you that you would like to change or improve. Really get a sense of what that issue feels like. **Ask** yourself, "What do I need to be aware of related to this issue?" Then, after you've asked, open this book to a random page.

The answer you are seeking should be somewhere on that page. Read as much as you need to satisfy your question. Afterward, you may notice that you feel lighter and less attached to your issue.

You can repeat this exercise two more times. Each time, you will go deeper with the harmonization of your issue.

Once you've received your third answer, you can trust that you're in the right place. Even better, just by asking those questions and receiving the answers, you've energetically harmonized yourself with everything else in the book. Your conscious mind, your subconscious mind, and your soul are aligned to help you get the most out of it, for your specific needs.

You don't want to just read this book. You want to be part of it, and you want it to be part of you. *That place of harmony and alignment is where your personal miracle begins to unfold.*

All You Have to Do Is Ask

Who knows you better than you do? No one.

Until now, you probably thought that the power to shift your health belonged to trained health practitioners. You've been following the same old medical traditions that people have been trudging through for years—covering up symptoms instead of eliminating them—because you thought it was the only thing you could do.

You've been thinking too much. Now, it's time to stop thinking and start feeling.

It's time to allow your personal connection to Source to be your guide.

It's true that you can't keep doing the same thing and expect to get a different result. This is an opportunity to try something new and walk a different path—one that is built for you, by you. The ability to sense and harmonize energy is in your hands, just by virtue of what you are. As simple and natural as it is, that ability also has the power to transform your health and your life.

Once you know how to harmonize energy, you'll find that you're not dependent on health practitioners anymore. You can use them as resources, if that's what your energy suggests, but you no longer have to accept everything they say as the last word. You are your own first and last word, and best of all, now you know how to read. No one can ever trump your internal truth, and nobody can treat you better than you can.

After everything you've been through and the countless specialists you've seen, the person who will finally fix your health issue once and for all is you yourself. Because at the end of the day, the truth is really incredibly simple: both the question and the answer to what you seek to change are already within you.

All you have to do is ask.

Chapter One:

OVERVIEW

Energy of You, for You

The method I've put together for working with energy is not a system. It's a set of tools for accessing and harmonizing the field of energy—specifically, yours.

The experience of this energy work is never the same for two people, because no two people are exactly the same. That's the way it's meant to be. You're meant to incorporate this modality into your individual life, for your individual needs, guided all the while by your personal connection to Source. You can come back to its principles again and again, and every time, you'll feel yourself going deeper.

My journey to working with energy has been exactly that: a deepening. As I mentioned earlier, I was born intuitive. That intuitive compass was the guide that led me to the work I do today.

My Path to Facilitating Energy: The Early Framework

My earliest framework for making sense out of my energetic abilities came in the form of religion.

As a toddler, I was naturally attuned to the field of energy around me. I could sense when my mother was worried or concerned, and I was able to comfort her just by being around her.

My intuition grew stronger as I got older. Because my biological father was not a part of my life, I was raised by my mother and stepfather. As a small child, I used to lie in bed looking up at the ceiling, wondering, "Why am I here? Why don't I have a father like everybody else?" My family was Catholic, and the answer that came back to me was, *Jesus is your father.*

That made sense to me. And when I went to church with my mother and grandmother and heard the priests talking about Jesus's healings, I thought, "Well, since he's my father, maybe I can do that, too." I didn't have an intention to heal at that point. I just took the idea for granted.

It wasn't until my holy communion that everything really came together.

That summer evening in first grade, my mother dressed me in a white shirt with a little tie, and I walked down the block with her and my stepfather to our local Catholic church. About twenty other kids were there with me at the church, both girls and boys. The priest guided us through the traditional ceremony. "You are going to receive the body of Christ," he said, "and you will be one with God."

Now, as a little kid, when people said things like that, I took them literally. *Okay, cool*, I thought. *Give it to me.*

And right there in that church, I did become one with God.

If you could have taken a picture of my aura at that moment, I would have been blinding. I *felt* the light—huge and glowing, both within and without. You want me to walk on water? Okay, no problem. You want me to float? Sure, I've done that. I aligned energetically with Christ. Those nights of staring at my ceiling as a four-year-old wondering "Why am I here?" matched up with my current experience. Christ *was* my father, and this—the enormous feeling of connection and awakening—*this* was my purpose.

I felt like I could fly. In fact, I kind of did fly home. My mother and stepfather had returned to our apartment after the ceremony, telling me that I could walk back a little later with the neighbors, because I wanted to hang out with the other kids for a bit first. But I didn't wait for the neighbors. I just took off running, out into the warm night, sprinting down the block like I had wings.

It was about half past nine at night, no one else around in our small California town. The desert sky was filled with a full moon and bright stars, and I followed them home like they were the star of Bethlehem itself, flying around the corner down the half-alley that led to the apartment, up the stairs, into my room.

When I got there, I was still on cloud nine. I threw off my little tie and did a somersault onto my bed, then planted myself upside down with my feet up against the wall and my head on my pillow. I stayed that way for a few minutes, just to calm my head.

I had tapped into my total perfected essence in Source, and I knew it. *Wow, that was amazing,* I thought. *That was exactly what was supposed to happen.*

I found it.

Psychic Dreams and Stolen Bike

After that, the clarity of my intuition snowballed.

I started to see things before they happened, usually in dreams. I had always had fairly psychic dreams, but now they seemed too frequent, too coincidental. And when it came to sharing them, I learned pretty quickly that it was better to say "I dreamt that something is going to happen to you" than "I saw that something is going to happen to you." Otherwise, my friends blamed me for the events when they turned out to be accurate.

One of my best friends, Simon, rode a bike to school. When we were in fifth grade, I had a dream that his bike would be stolen if he brought it to school the next day. So I warned him to leave it at home. Simon shook his head. "Hector, I know you told me that other things have come true in your dreams, but I live far away. My parents aren't going to bring me here, and there's no bus that goes by my house. I'll just lock up the bike."

Simon rode the bike to school. And sure enough, late the next afternoon, he came looking for me. "Hey Hector, where's my bike?" he demanded.

The bike was gone, and he thought that I'd taken it on purpose to prove a point.

Of course I hadn't taken it, but I could feel the energy of where the bike had been taken. I helped Simon track it down about two miles from the school, in somebody's carport. The kids who had taken it were gang members, and they had already painted the bike to cover their tracks, but it still had a serial number. We called the cops and got it back. All Simon had to do was repaint it.

My "dreams" weren't limited to sleeping hours. I could also intuit things that I needed while I was awake—something that came in handy for taking tests at school. The teacher would say, "On Friday, we're going to have a test on these three chapters." Well, I didn't want to study every word of those three chapters. I wanted to study exactly what she wanted me to focus on. So I tapped into which parts of those three chapters I really needed to know for the test, and I did well on the exam.

"I think you're cheating," teachers said to me once in a while.

"No, I'm not. I'm just reading your mind," I told them. And they left me alone after that, because nobody believed that such a thing was possible.

Cross-Country Harmony

My first really focused attempt to help other people with my abilities was directed at my high school cross-country team.

By now, I was beginning to discover parallels for the energetic abilities I had in areas beyond my Catholic upbringing, such as Hatha yoga and meditation. I put these tools to work not just for myself as a cross-country participant, but also for the other members of my team and for the younger kids I coached.

The night before each competition, I meditated. I visualized the course through remote viewing, running through it in my mind and testing my time at each benchmark. Then I did the same for each of the other runners.

The next day, I told them what I'd seen.

I explained who would cross the finish line in what order, and what each person's time would be. They knew me well enough to trust what I told them. "Look," I said, "all you have to do is run free. Just like the wind. Be effortless."

That harmonized the energetic field of the team. Each person used the information I gave him to tap into his own innate intelligence and create the best-case scenario I'd seen. Every time, they ran their best race. And sure enough, we won consistently—all the way up to the championship.

"Wow," our coach told me in amazement, "you're a great motivator. I hope you become a track and field coach after you graduate."

"I'm Gonna Marry That Girl"

I knew that I would marry my wife the day I met her in our high school chemistry class.

Simon was in that class with me, and that day we were doing a lab assignment, mixing up some chemicals. We were just going along, following the steps, when our experiment exploded.

Everyone in the class turned and stared at us. I thought for sure we were in trouble, but I was wrong. "You got the perfect thermodynamic reaction!" our teacher clapped. "Great work!"

Great work or not, the explosion still made a mess. So I went to the janitor's closet to get some cleaning supplies. On my way to put them back, I passed a couple of girls who were having trouble with their experiment. "Hey, do you need help?" I asked them. They said sure, so I told them how to get their experiment to work. Then I went back to my desk and sat down next to Simon.

"See that girl over there?" I asked him, nodding at one of the girls I'd just helped. I barely knew who she was. "I'm going to marry her."

"Oh, you're always saying things," Simon said, blowing me off.

And we just went back to what we were doing.

Vows

A few years later, I went to a New Year's Eve party and met up with the girl from my high school class again. We hit it off, and we kept in touch for several months before we actually started dating. At that time, I was attending medical school, but when I clairvoyantly saw that my university was taking me in a different direction than I needed to go, I asked my then-girlfriend for advice about changing directions.

"What do you want to be when you grow up?" she asked me.

I knew I wanted to be in the health field—some kind of holistic doctor. So I switched schools, did my undergraduate degree, and finally made it into the celebrated Los Angeles College of Chiropractic. I asked my wife to marry me before I started the program, and she came with me.

I always used my intuitive abilities to expand on the physical work I did with patients during and after college, no matter where I was working. But my resolve to develop my own methodology for facilitating healing energy was sparked by a personal tragedy.

In the early 2000s, my wife and I had a daughter whom we lost shortly after her birth.

Her death was the result of a misstep in her care by the hospital where we were staying. The deep anger, frustration, and loss of that experience made clear to me the path I needed to take. I vowed to do everything I could not just to make sure that no one else had to go through what we went through, but to find a way to improve the universe from this event. The work I was doing with clinics and other energy facilitators—and even the basic work I had been doing on my own since 1988—was no longer enough.

I had to create a more effective way of bringing the awareness of energy work to the world.

Between 2002 and 2008, I began to develop my original energy work into a more structured, powerful methodology. Slowly, I transitioned away from working within the limitations of other people's systems, all the while continuing to do my own thing. In 2008, I finished structuring my method, Garcia Innergetics. My evolved method was effortless—and reproducible.

In 2010, I felt it was time to share Garcia Innergetics with the world.

You: A Toolbox for Health

Thousands of people have seen positive results from the energy method you're about to embark on in these chapters. But you need to understand that my way of working with energy is not a system. It's not a predetermined, step-by-step set of instructions for constructing perfect health. Why?

Because you are unique unto yourself, day to day and moment by moment.

You're also the keeper of your own individual blueprint for well-being. When you look at it from this angle, you can see that no modality can be a cookie-cutter set of instructions that will be exactly right for everyone. We're not meant to work that way.

But I *can* give you tools, and I can show you how to use the resources available to you so that you can apply them to your personal blueprint.

From there, you can build anything you want in your life—including good health.

All of this begs the question: What are the tools you need to commence work on your blueprint?

What is energy? To work effectively with energy, you first need to understand what it is. I consider energy to be the source of everything. When you connect to it, you have access to its knowledge, and it can tell you exactly what's going on.

Stop thinking; start feeling. One of the biggest obstacles to accessing the power of energy is our minds. Energy is self-intelligent, but that doesn't mean it follows our logic. Far from it. When you learn to stop thinking and notice how you feel, you open the path to receive the answers you're looking for.

Tap into your GPS. Your Guided Personal Source, or GPS, holds the exact information you need at any given time. The key is learning to tap into it using the powerful tools of intention, knowingness, and neutrality.

Maintain energetic balance and navigate the morphic field. Energy is always in flux. Even after you harmonize your energy using your GPS, your health can still be affected by triggers in the environment around you, such as people, situations, or the weather. These environmental conditions can be part of the morphic field. When you learn to move through it with neutrality, you empower yourself to maintain energetic balance.

Approach common health issues with an energetic view. Not every health condition is caused by the same thing in all individuals. If you have a heart condition, it doesn't have to follow that you're a heavyset male with high cholesterol. Many health issues have emotional roots, or come from off the body altogether. I've had success resolving myriad health problems with energy, including addictions, AIDS, Alzheimer's and dementia, asthma, autism, autoimmune disorders, cancer, cerebral palsy, colds and bronchial infections, diabetes, heart disease (including blood pressure and cholesterol), hypertension, infertility, Lyme disease and Morgellons, multiple sclerosis, nervous disorders, obesity, renal failure, vertigo, and vision issues. The more open minded you are about the source of your health condition, the better you'll be able to receive the information you need.

Harmonize energy beyond your health. Everything is energy, and energy is everything. That includes your health, but it's far from limited to it. You can use this same set of tools to energetically improve any area of your life, including money, finance, occupation, career, relationships, and future and life purpose.

Remember that you and Source are one. All energy comes from Source, and that includes you. You are a small hologram of the infinite whole, and you can connect to it. You truly have access to everything out there. Once you recognize that, you can take your ability to harmonize energy to very powerful heights.

Garcia Innergetics is not designed to give you line-by-line instructions on working with energy. It's designed to teach you to read *between* the lines, using personal Source as your guide. When you connect to the spiritual part of yourself without limited expectations about the answers you "should" receive, you will discover things that you never imagined you would find, things that have the power to transform your life into whatever you want it to be.

In the chapters that follow, I will share stories of individuals who have used Garcia Innergetics to effect this kind of transformation for themselves. The details of these particular case studies—including the names of clients and their case specifics—have been changed to protect the privacy of those involved.

Once you have the right tools, all of the possibilities and probabilities that the energy has to offer will be at your fingertips. And all of that begins with the most basic tool in the box: understanding what energy really is.

Chapter Two:

WHAT IS ENERGY?

The Tumor Is Gone

A regular client of mine, Alma, called me up one day with some concerning news. She was experiencing uterine bleeding. "Should I come see you or go to my OB/GYN first?" she asked.

I told her to go see her OB/GYN first and then come see me, which is protocol in cases like this. So Alma scheduled an appointment with her doctor that same morning. They gave her an ultrasound and an MRI. Then they told her to come back later that afternoon after the images came back so that they could go over the results with her.

In the meantime, Alma came into my office during the lunch hour to get my take on the issue. I connected with her energy. "Yeah, there's something there," I confirmed. It was coming from off the body, in a different level of energy—a parallel universe. I tracked the level down, matched the pattern there with her tumor, and inverted the energetic field.

Immediately, she sensed a shift in energy in her lower abdomen.

Alma thanked me and went back to her doctor to hear the report of findings from her tests. I went back to my regular work schedule. Then, late in the afternoon, she came back to the office with a look of awestruck surprise on her face. I was with another client, so she told the whole story to my assistant at the front desk. "It's gone!" she announced. "Is that normal?"

The MRI from that morning had shown a large mass in her uterus. However, when she returned to see the doctor, he palpated the area and nothing was there. "That doesn't make sense," he said, and he went to get a second doctor. The second doctor was just as perplexed and brought in a third doctor, who couldn't figure it out either. "Maybe the MRI belongs to a different patient? Maybe the names got mixed up?" they guessed. But when they went to double check, the MRI really was Alma's. In the end, there was nothing to do but send her home.

Alma's tumor had dissolved in the space of a lunch break. Not because of me.

It dissolved because she connected with the energy field to allow the change to take place.

Everything Is Energy, and Energy Is Everything

What is energy?

The simple answer to this question is: everything. Everything is energy, and energy is everything. The how, why, when, and what of your situation—how it feels, why you came to have it, when it occurred—is encoded within energy itself. That's why, once you know how to read it, you can work with it to change your outcomes. This concept lies at the heart of *Guiding Personal Source*.

The life force of everything stems from the field of energy. But how do we identify life force?

I like to look at this using Einstein's definition of energy as $E = mc^2$.

In my clairvoyant awareness, E equals "expression of spirit." Everything has spirit, and everything is united through spirit. The m stands for "mindful mission." This is the intent you have to change and harmonize the field of energy. The first c stands for "consciousness"—your awareness that something could be better. And the second c equals "connection," meaning that you are connected to what is in your best interest.

Even if you break down the simple physics and chemistry of it, everything leads back to the spark of spirit that keeps things running. Energy is the source of spirit itself.

You might be thinking, "All right, Garcia, but if I'm made of energy, why isn't that obvious to me? Why do I feel like a solid, lumpy body surrounded by hard physical things?"

Think of it this way. Say you have a pool, and you're about to go swimming. Before you start, you're acclimated to the temperature of the air around you, and you feel comfortable. Then you jump in the water. The temperature of the water is colder, and at first you feel a sharp difference between it and you. Then, after you've been in the pool for a while, that sensation changes. You acclimate to the temperature of the water, and soon you can't really feel a separation between that water and your body anymore.

That's the flow of energy at work, and it's not limited to swimming pools. The dense physical body you've acclimated to *is* a frequency of energy. But it's not the only frequency you're working with.

You are a spiritual being having a mind-body experience. You've become used to the physical, maybe to the point where you've lost touch with the spiritual sense of yourself. However, that doesn't change the nature of what you are, or the fact that you can retune your awareness to and shift energy beyond the physical level.

You just need to acknowledge all the possibilities of who and what you are.

This chapter will walk you through the basics of energy, which goes both ways, has its own logic, and manifests in fields. I'll also show you why, using this method of energy work, you cannot cause harm to yourself or anyone else— only harmony.

Energy Goes Both Ways

A key concept to understand about energy is that it goes both ways.

Energy is multidirectional. As soon as you connect with an energy pattern, it is also connecting with you. For example, if you have a migraine, then you are thinking about that migraine, and the migraine is thinking about you.

This isn't limited to health issues. If I'm thinking about my cat, my cat is also thinking about me. If I'm thinking about my car, my car is thinking about me, too.

Everything has directional force because everything is energy, and everything exists in an energetic relationship with everything else. This is known as quantum entanglement, first identified by Albert Einstein in the early 1900s. Einstein called it "Spooky Action at a Distance" or "Quantum Weirdness." While energy is multidirectional, we experience it as mostly going in the direction of the observer. You can think of yourself as the hub at the center of a wheel, with energy bombarding you from many different spokes at once.

Now, that said, energy is never "out to get you."

Even though energy goes both ways, you are never a victim of energy. Many people create a victim mentality for themselves by holding on to their issues. However, that's just a state of mind. You always have the power to become aware of the energetic conditions around you. As soon as you're aware of those conditions, you have the ability to deal with them.

Energy is never malevolent. It works through a system of positive and negative polarities, but energy itself is neutral. Why then do we hear people talking about "good energy" and "bad energy"?

This is where the role of free will comes into play.

You have the direct ability to transform or manifest what your mind intends. If you want to believe energy is bad, then you can move it in that direction. At the same time, energy has an equal and infinite capacity to be used in a positive way.

Because energy goes both ways, your health issue itself has will much like you do. However, the difference is that the will of the field around you—including your health condition—is opportunistic.

For example, if you have migraines, you probably have them because you're the perfect host and you're not really willing to let go of the issue—even though you might consciously think you are.

A lot of people have trouble with this idea. "How can you say that my free will is keeping me sick?" they say. "I don't *want* to be sick."

In cases like these, the individuals have allowed their minds to take over their free will. Mentally, they don't support the idea of letting their issues go. *The mind is a terrible thing to use, unless you control it.* You control it by allowing the awareness to grow that you do have the power of free will, and by being neutral to your situation. I'll explain more about the energetic tool of neutrality in chapters 3 and 4.

Energy work is very powerful, but it cannot override your free will. You have the freedom to hold on to your issue or let it go, to support the change or resist it.

The choice is always yours.

Energy Has Its Own Logic

In addition to going both ways, energy is also self-intelligent.

By "intelligent," I'm not talking about logic in the way our minds understand it. Energy is not logical in the way we think about logic. The opposite is true. It has its own logic, which works along the lines of what is known as an energetic relationship.

In an energetic relationship, energy exists between two fields. These fields encompass infinite information, which you are able to access using your intuition. Your intent acts as the first point, and the information you're accessing is the second point. That information can be anywhere in the field. Once you make that connection, the energetic field makes the information available to you.

For example, our idea of logic goes something like, "If X, then Y, in a linear fashion." Energy's idea of logic might be something along the lines of, "If X, then G—right now. But P three minutes from now. Oh look, another alphabet; let's go there." And the amazing thing is, working by its own idea of logic, it always comes up with the optimal result.

"Logic" from an energetic perspective means that energy doesn't follow one set path. It's open to every possibility— even the ones beyond the grasp of the human mind. Dean Radin identified this phenomenon as Random Generator in 1989. His experiments measured global and group consciousness and concluded that energy has many possibilities. That's why it can give you all kinds of information that you never could have discovered using the limitations of manmade logic. And that's one of the reasons energy is so powerful.

For example, you may assume that you have your health issue for a certain "logical" reason. To go back to the migraine example, let's say you have a friend who gets migraines from drinking caffeine. You think to yourself, "Oh, I also drink caffeine. That must be why I have migraines, too."

That assumption isn't true. The cause of your migraines could be literally anything. It may be the reason you have in mind, but it could also be anything else. And it's usually something else.

Because of its innate intelligence, the energy is able to match up to whatever that "something else" is as soon as you ask the question. It offers you the information you need, and you can allow the resulting energetic transformation to harmonize the field from there.

Energy Fields

When I say "harmonize the field," what field am I talking about?

In physics, a field is created when two or more points connect. An energy field is the energetic flow of information. Even though energy is multidirectional, it expresses itself in patterns. You yourself are a field of energy. Energy flows through you in a unique way that makes you identifiable as you.

For example, if you're in the ocean, which ocean are you in? All oceans are connected, but the energy of the Pacific

Ocean is completely different from the energy of the Atlantic Ocean, and the energy of the Atlantic Ocean is different from that of the Indian Ocean.

You can feel an energy field right now. Take your hands and hold them so that the palms are facing each other, about one inch apart. The heat and tension you notice happening between them is a form of subtle energy. In his book *Life Source*, prominent physicist Claude Swanson defines subtle energy as a bridge between energy fields.

The goal is to keep yourself in harmony as an energy field among energy fields, all of which are in a constant state of motion.

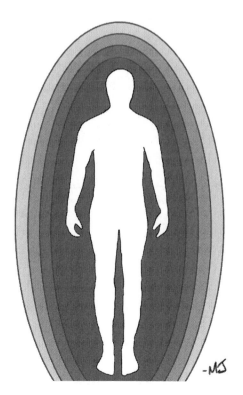

There are twenty-two different energy fields that I teach to my students in my courses. Five of them are macrocosmic, ten are intrinsic, and seven are microcosmic. Macrocosmic energy fields exist at a large-scale universal level. Intrinsic energy fields include the physical, mental, and emotional aspects of our existence, such as acupuncture meridians, chakras, and the astral body. Microcosmic fields refer to things such as molecular energy and quantum entanglement. Your health issue may be coming from any of these different fields. However, you don't need to identify each of them by name when you're doing this work, because the energy itself is intelligence. It already understands these fields, even if you don't.

Because that's the case, it will bring you the outcome you ask for from whichever field has the answer. You have the option of going deeper into the work and connecting to specific fields if you want to. But for the purposes of this book, you don't have to know the specifics of where the answer came from to experience the results. And that makes the whole method very accessible to anyone and everyone.

No Harm, Just Harmony

Anyone can work with energy. That includes you.

Remember, energy is everything, and everything is energy. You are energy, and you're about to tap into the tools that will allow you to start accessing that natural state of being. You'll use those tools your way, tapping into the field in a manner that feels right to you. But as long as you understand how energy flows, you have the power to harmonize it.

It doesn't matter if you've had previous experience working with energy or not. In fact, if you have no experience, you'll probably see faster success, because you're a blank canvas. You don't have to grapple with the mental limitations of other energy systems you've dealt with in the past. And if you do have previous experience, don't worry; all is not lost. You're just going to have to train yourself to be neutral to the other modalities you've learned in the past, such as Reiki, acupuncture, and others.

The fewer regulations your mind has about how energy "should" work, the more powerful you become—simply because you're open to the information that is coming to you, whatever it might be.

People sometimes ask me, "Okay, but just because I *can* work with energy doesn't mean I'm going to do it right. What if I screw it up?"

The answer is simple: using this method, you can't.

You can't, because rather than being a healer, you are just a facilitator of healing energy, working in harmony with it. This is one of the things that makes Garcia Innergetics unique. Garcia Innergetics is not about controlling energy. It's about letting the energy bring you information, and then harmonizing the field. Remember, energy is self-intelligent, and it has access to everything. When you ask it a question, it knows what needs to be done, and it brings you that knowledge. The only thing that shows up is exactly what needs to be harmonized.

You don't need to decide what's right and wrong. The energy already knows. That means that you are guaranteed to walk the right path every time, because you're not assuming anything. You're never going against the harmony of energetic flow. You can't. The energy won't allow you to. This is why working with energy is safe and accessible.

Energy Is Infinite

Energy is difficult to understand in its totality by the very nature of what it is, because it is infinite. It's always shifting. Even the pure energy that responds to us specifically, as our guiding personal Source, is really beyond our comprehension, because it reacts in ways that our minds can never fully capture or make sense of. The more you work with energy, the more you find that it refuses to match up to your mental limitations.

That sets us up for one of the biggest obstacles to working with energy: thinking.

In the next chapter, I'll show you how to stop thinking and start feeling your way to improved health.

Chapter Three:

STOP THINKING; START FEELING

The Shift

When I teach my classes, I can always feel the shift in my students when they stop thinking and start feeling, as clear as day and night.

They walk into the room with all kinds of different emotions, and each of them is searching for something different. Some are looking for personal growth, some are there to enhance their intuition, and others are spiritual healers hoping to learn additional tools to help with their practice. Most are excited to learn and explore their potential. However, one thing that sometimes stands between them and their ability to tap into those areas, is that they often start out more connected to mind than Source.

So prior to teaching the class, I condition the space. I do this by having them tap into their intention for being in attendance. This creates a morphic field specifically for them, paving the way for a shift. I have them activate their pineal gland, which helps them become one with Source. Then I lead them through a meditation.

"Close your eyes," I say, and they do. "Take a deep breath in. Now, bring your attention to your center, to your heart. Focus on something that you want to work on. Go beneath the thought of the issue that's bothering you. Notice how that feels." I pause to let them get a really good feel for it. Then I continue. "Breathe in the issue, and breathe it out. Release it. That issue is gone. Now center yourself in your lower belly. This is where you're going to receive and install the information I'm going to share with you this weekend.

"Open your eyes."

They open their eyes. Any uncertainty, apprehension, or preconceived ideas that they came in with are gone. Instead, they look at me with hope, peace, and focus. Already, they feel lighter, united in a sacred space. They're more open to what I'm about to teach them, because they're not thinking anymore. Instead, they're feeling. They are truly receptive and ready to learn.

And we begin.

Prepare the Ground

A major tool in the Garcia Innergetics method of working with energy as your Guiding Personal Source is to stop thinking and start feeling.

There's a famous saying that goes, "I think, therefore I am." The speaker should have added two more words to the end of that sentence: "I think, therefore I am messed up." Our minds are very restrictive, because thinking comes with filters in the form of references from the past, which some consider to be cell memory. When you spend your time constantly thinking, you limit the ability of the field to function effectively.

It's like opening Pandora's Box. You fixate on one thought, and the issue snowballs. "Okay, if I do this, the outcome will be that. But if I do that, the outcome will be something else. Maybe if I don't do anything the outcome will be in my favor. But then again, maybe not . . ."

The more you dwell in this thinking process, the more problems and chaos you put into your energy field. Imagine the flow of energy like a road. Thinking throws orange cones and potholes into your road, and those obstacles block answers from coming to you.

Feeling is just the opposite.

When you feel, you are connecting to universal awareness itself, and it connects to you. You're not just conscious, because consciousness is limiting. You can be conscious of being aware, but you can't be aware of being conscious. Awareness, which I call "knowingness," is intuitive, flexible, and pliable. To feel is to truly step into your full sense of awareness.

47

Once you stop thinking about your issue and just notice how it feels—not how you feel about it, but how it truly feels—that gives you a direction for harmonizing the energy. It clears your road and sets up a field where information can come to you freely. Some people refer to this as a "gut feeling."

When you put yourself in touch with how you feel about your issue, you are getting the true essence of what it is, and the energy will be able to guide you to where you need to go next. The more you insist on thinking, the more difficult it will be to move forward and let go.

Letting go is a very hard thing to do for a lot of people. Even though in their conscious minds they think they want to get better, their *subconscious* minds are afraid of change. The subconscious may equate change with death. So they keep holding on to their issues, because even though they're unhappy, they feel comfortable in what they know, as opposed to what is unknown to them.

Learning to stop thinking and start feeling gives you the courage to let go and move on. The more you feel, the more you allow the field of energy to help, guide, and protect you on your way to better health. This chapter will show you how to release your ego, embrace knowingness, and prepare the ground for harmonization by tapping into your ability to feel.

Effortlessly Egoless

Most of us are our own biggest obstacle to working with energy effectively. That internal obstacle is usually an ego issue.

Thinking and ego go hand in hand. I define ego as E.G.O.: energy going out. All of us have ego. The problem occurs when we don't control how much of our energy is going out.

Control is a key issue when it comes to ego. We recklessly exercise our egos because we imagine that sending out a lot of energy means being in control. Having one up on someone else makes us think we're in control. Believing that we're the source of creating things makes us think we're in control.

In reality, nothing could be further from the truth.

Just because we're sending energy out doesn't mean that that energy output is effective. All it means is that we're giving our minds something to do—something to think about. As soon as that happens and we spiral into a thinking pattern, we actually *lose* control of ourselves, and our egos take over.

You never want that to happen, especially when you're facilitating energy. Instead, you want to hold on to control by going within your heart space. There, you can allow yourself to feel the love in the universe flowing to you through the fields of energy in and around you.

True control is letting go. It's entering a state of feeling neutral, unattached. If you allow the energy to just be, you can never have excess ego, because there's no place for it to grow. Instead of energy going out, you have energy coming in, in the form of intuition, love, and awareness. The less you think, the less ego you have, and the more bandwidth you have to feel the energy.

You become effortlessly egoless. And that's right where you want to be.

Stop Thinking; Start Feeling

Now you understand why it's so important to leave your mind behind and embrace your intuition. So how do you actually stop thinking and start feeling?

When I say "stop thinking," I don't literally mean "stop your thoughts from existing." Instead, I want you to stop taking them so seriously. Don't worry about them. Let them pass through without seizing upon them in transit and building a lot of preconceived notions. Once you can do this, all the space you used to dedicate to thinking will open up, and feeling will step in to fill that void naturally.

Try this exercise to help yourself transition out of thinking and into feeling.

Exercise: Center Yourself

One of the best ways to move into a state of feeling is simply to move your focus from your mind to your center. At your center, you are a divine creation of Source. You have no doubt and no worries—no reason to think and every reason to feel. Here are a few exercises to shift yourself to a centered state of awareness.

- **Picture your heart.** Close your eyes and allow your focus to settle on your center, at your heart chakra or breastbone. Breathe in and out from that point of knowingness a few times.

- **Lace your fingers.** Bring your hands together with interlaced fingers, and notice which thumb is on top—the right one or the left. Then, separate your hands and re-lace your fingers, putting the non-dominant thumb on top. Doing this about ten times balances your left and right brain.

- **Touch your tongue to the roof of your mouth.** Press the tip of your tongue to the roof of your mouth, and stand with your toes straight or slightly pigeon-toed for a little while. This brings in energy that gives you a sense of balance and calm focus. I believe that this is a way of connecting with your total essence—a form of and a pathway to Source.

An Avenue of Possibilities

Learning to let go of your mind is one of the most fundamental tools in the Garcia Innergetics toolbox. Once you truly allow your mind to let go, you are no longer confined by mental limitations or trapped in a box of outdated beliefs. You're in touch with your guiding personal Source, and you are free. You've cleared out the old, and now you have room for a whole avenue of possibilities that you weren't aware of before.

You can create whatever you want, including a more positive outcome for your health. All you need to do is harmonize the energy. In the next chapter, I'll show you how to do that by tapping into your "GPS"—Guided Personal Source—itself, using intention, knowingness, and neutrality.

Chapter Four:

TAP INTO YOUR GPS

An Unexpected Event

Mary was forty-eight years old when she came to see me for a consultation regarding a cancer diagnosis. Her diagnosis was recent, and she wanted to proceed with the regular medical route as well as working with me to make sure that she covered both her allopathic and holistic bases.

I tested her energy field and said, "Perfect. Both treatments will complement each other in your case. Let's go for it."

I worked with Mary once a month for about a year, and the doctors were so amazed by how fast she recovered that they actually forgot to schedule checkups for her after a while. Meanwhile, during our time together, Mary learned that she could also use energy to improve areas of life beyond her health. After the cancer had been eradicated, she continued seeing me for help with her business, coming in for regular appointments.

One day, she walked in the door and I could tell that something was different. I asked her what was new in her life.

Her eyes went as big as saucers. "Why?" she asked. "Who told you about it?"

"What?" I said. "Nobody told me anything. I just sensed something different in your energy."

Mary looked at me and said, "I just found out I'm pregnant."

Then she told me her whole story. She had wanted children for years, and she'd tried everything to make it happen, including in vitro fertilization (IVF). When the IVF started to take a toll on her other health issues, she'd been forced to stop undergoing it. She'd completely given up hope of ever getting pregnant.

"This changes my whole outlook on life and my business," Mary admitted.

"Well, business can wait, but this baby can't," I told her. "Let's harmonize the energy so that he's perfect when he gets here."

Mary gave birth to a healthy baby boy several months later—still stunned, but very happy to have the child she'd always wanted at last.

What Is Guided Personal Source (GPS)?

I facilitated the energy that shifted Mary's cancer and harmonized her fertility, but I wasn't the one who made those outcomes happen. All I did was connect with the place within Mary that already knew what needed to be done: her Guided Personal Source.

Guided Personal Source, or GPS, is a key part of facilitating energy. It really is your personal energy map. Your GPS is both the keeper of the answers you need and the tool you use to allow the part of you that is Source to guide you to the personalized outcomes you want—or, more accurately, to guide the information you need to you. The answers it brings you belong to you and no one else. If you have migraines, your GPS will tell you what the source of *your* migraines are, regardless of what the medical books say or why everyone else gets headaches.

The concept of Guided Personal Source has been demonstrated by various experiments. Lynne McTaggart, author of *The Intention Experiment*, conducted research validating that information is self-encoded in our cells. Gary E. Schwartz, PhD, director of the Laboratory for Advances in Consciousness and Health at Arizona State University, demonstrated in his book *The Energy Healing Experiments* that individuals who receive heart transplants often take on the characteristics of the heart's previous owner as a result of cell memory. For example, an individual who never had trouble sleeping before her transplant developed insomnia soon afterward, only to learn that her heart had come from a night watchman.

Accessing your GPS allows you to identify the answers you've been looking for. But more than that, it's also the tool you use to fix things once you have those answers.

Taking action to harmonize the energy once it shows you what needs to be done is one of the things that makes this method of energy work unique. Clients come to me all the time saying, "Oh, I got a bad reading from my astrologer," or "My tarot reader said that I'm going to experience a calamity in my life." When I ask them what the astrologer or the tarot reader did about it, the clients tell me, "Well, nothing. They just gave me the information."

Most of the time, I'll test the situation, and then I'll say, "Yes, your astrologer was right. Now, let's fix it." I connect into the client's GPS, harmonize the field, and shift the information he or she was given. That's the true power of working with energy. If you don't like the answers you get, you can change them.

Your GPS is both your energetic signature and your guide as a facilitator of that energy. You are your own energy facilitator, and your GPS will tell you everything you need to know to work with your own powerful field of energy effectively. With this method, you never impose your will to create outcomes. The energy itself is the transformer, regulating and refining the energy field of your body. In this chapter, I'll teach you the foundational principles that support your GPS and show you how to use this powerful energetic tool.

The Foundation: Intention, Knowingness, Neutrality

The concept of GPS works on three key principles: intention, knowingness, and neutrality.

Before you can use your GPS effectively, you need to establish a strong, clear relationship with each of these three things. Each of them is a tool in your energetic toolbox in and of itself. You can think of them as critical parts of a car. If your car is completely built except for the steering wheel, you're not going anywhere. The same is true for the wheels, or the engine. Once you understand intention, knowingness, and neutrality, you are in a position to turn the car on and drive.

Let's look at each of these fundamental concepts one at a time.

Intention

Intention is simply your desire to create, do, or accomplish something.

The reason intention is so powerful is that it begins the process of change. It starts the car moving in a specific direction. Without intention, nothing is ever going to get started in the first place, and you'll never reach an end result. Renowned physicist William Tiller proved this in his experiments on subtle energy in the early 2000s, in which he demonstrated that intention could imprint a measurable effect on electronic devices.

Imagine that you're going on a trip to a new destination, driving from one place to another. The first thing you do is track your route in Google maps to help you get from point A to point B. If you don't input your "to" and "from" locations to begin with, you won't know where to go, and you'll never be guided to the specific place you want to reach.

Intention works the same way. If you want to create something, you have to start somewhere. Often, we aren't clear on what we should do before we do it. In that case, intention takes the form of a simple question. Asking your energy what the best course of action is for you gives you a starting point, because your intent itself has self-intelligence. As soon as you form it, it knows where to go. The intention itself causes a shift to correct the situation.

You can have any answer you want, as long as you're willing to ask for it. That's the true power of intention.

Knowingness

Like intention, knowingness has self-intelligence. It's the awareness you have within yourself that directs you to the right course of action to take. Some people think of this as the intuition, which gives you a "gut feeling."

Knowingness does not mean that you know everything with your conscious mind. Knowingness is the awareness that you don't *have* to know it all. The only thing you have to know is that the answer exists somewhere, in some energetic plane of existence. When you have knowingness, you are really inviting the answers to come to you, rather than you going out in search of the answers.

Knowingness is the alpha and the omega, the beginning and the end. I know the end because I know the beginning. I know the beginning because there is an end. I don't trust. I go beyond trust.

The reason I make a distinction between knowingness and trust is that trust comes with the polarity of doubt. If you trust something, you also open up the possibility of doubting it. That throws you back into the trap of thinking instead of feeling.

But if you have knowingness, there is no room for doubt. As I tell my clients, "There's nothing to worry about, because the energy itself gave me the answer you're asking for." It's like reverse engineering. The end result gives you the answer, and therefore you always have the knowingness that the answer itself is right.

Try this exercise to tap into your sense of knowingness: Speak aloud the words, "I am happy." Notice how that feels to you.

Now, just say the word "happy." Feel this, too.

Once you're done with the exercise, compare the two. You should notice a difference between them. When you say, "I am happy," that sounds good, but at the same time you have the question "Why should I be happy?" lurking in your mind.

When you just say, "Happy," there is no question. There is only the sense of happiness, pure and simple. Nobody can block that feeling in you—not even your mind. It's a done deal, because it is part of your true perfected essence.

When you use phrases that have an opposite equivalent, it opens the door for doubt and thinking. If you speak only the word you want to feel, you access the true feeling of the word from a state of knowingness.

Remember, energy goes both ways. Once you get a sense of a feeling, that feeling also has you. And it can pull you in the direction you want to go.

Never buy in to the idea of "faith over doubt." Instead, hold a knowingness that what you're feeling is the truth, and the answers you receive will never steer you wrong.

Neutrality

The last core principle behind GPS is neutrality. Neutrality means that you have no attachment to the end result.

At first it sounds like a paradox. You begin with the intention to get a result, and then you have knowingness that the result will come to you. You're undertaking the work in the first place because you want a specific outcome.

So it seems counterintuitive and even ironic that, in order to actually get that result you're looking for, you ultimately have to release your attachment to it. But the reality is that, when you practice neutrality, you are actually going beyond both intention and knowingness. The moment you do, you get yourself out of the way, and your original intention and knowingness are free to bring you exactly what you asked for in the first place.

Neutrality can be the hardest principle to embrace in working with energy, because it means letting go. But when you do push past your attachment to a specific outcome, you become limitless. And limitless things can come to you—including the very thing you want.

Pilot Your GPS (with ASK)

Once you are connected to intention, knowingness, and neutrality, the work is already done. The only thing left to do is facilitate the energy. You're ready to pilot your GPS, using a tool I call ASK.

ASK stands for "assess, scan or connect, know." It creates a sacred openness of awareness for receiving information or transformation, and it is designed to allow you to test your energy using the guiding principles of intention, knowingness, and neutrality, so that the answers come to you instead of you going to the answers.

Picture a dog standing at the edge of a lake, and a bone floating in the middle of the water. The dog wants to get the bone. If he starts paddling to the middle of the lake (energy going out, or ego), he makes waves and the bone drifts away from him. But if he stands on the shore and waits, the currents of the water will bring the bone to him naturally.

We are using energy in a similar way when we ASK—only with much faster results. ASK is really the verb form of intention, knowingness, and neutrality. When you assess, you are tapping into your intention by asking a question. When you scan, you are accessing knowingness by finding the answer to the question. And when you know, you are moving into a state of neutrality and allowing the answer to come to you.

At the end of this process, the energy harmonizes itself naturally. There is nothing left that you need to do, because everything is already taken care of. You can feel the harmonization taking effect, usually as a sense of lightness or a faint buzz in your body.

Now that you know the concept, what does the physical act of ASKing look like?

How to ASK

When you first begin to work with energy, the easiest way to assess, scan, and know is usually by doing what appears to be a muscle test.

In actuality, you are not doing a muscle test. You are doing an energy test, and it looks very similar to muscle testing. In muscle testing, you have polarities: a positive pole and a negative one. Usually, if the answer you're looking for is "yes," the muscle is strong. If the muscle is weak, the answer is "no."

In energy testing, we use this process more like a dowsing rod. In our case, when you ask the right question, the muscle actually weakens to let you know you're on the right track. We are looking for an energetic entry to the issue we want to solve, and the testing makes it easy for us to see the entry. As soon as your muscle gives you a response to your question, you've accessed and identified the energy of the issue and shifted it.

Two common types of energy tests are arm tests and O-ring tests. Take a look at the examples of these in figure 4.1.

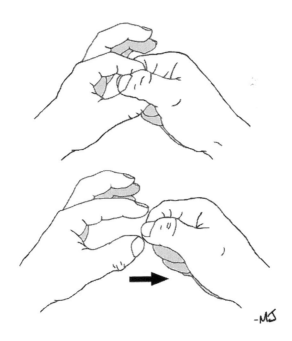

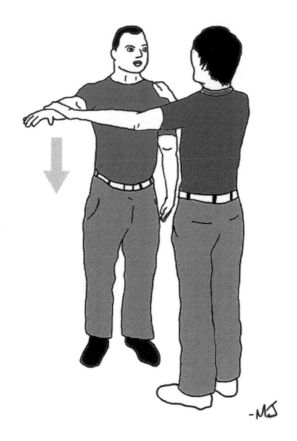

-MJ

Either one of these forms of testing will work. The arm test takes up space and works well if you're at home. The O-ring test is useful because you can do it anywhere—for example, on public transportation—without causing a scene.

Let's walk through the stages of ASK using an O-ring energy test.

Assess. Before you form your O-ring, you need to form your question. The question is directed at the issue you want to assess.

Here are three basic questions you can ask during an energy test:

1. *Is my issue really an issue?* Or, as we phrase it in my classes, "Issue, no issue?" Just because you have migraines doesn't mean that the migraines themselves are actually the source of the problem. In fact, more often than not, the issue stems from other things.

2. *Does thinking about my issue make it an issue?* Often, just thinking about an issue is what triggers the issue to take place. The problem isn't the issue itself. The problem is the thinking.

3. *Is the thought of* not *having an issue the problem?* This is very common. Sometimes, we want to have issues that we don't actually have, often just to give ourselves something to do. The subconscious part of us is thinking, "Hey, my mom has migraines. Why not me? I want to be special, too." This is considered reverse perception.

Scan. Once you have a question in mind, test it using the O-ring. Press your thumb and index finger together so that they form an O shape. Hold your fingertips together firmly, but not with so much strength that you're completely unmovable. Then press the thumb and index finger of your opposite hand together, also, and push them into the O-ring so that the thumbs are resting against each other and the index fingers are doing the same, as shown in figure 4.1.

Now, ask one of the three questions. Right after you ask the question, put pressure on the O-ring by separating the two fingers on the inside of it like a pair of tongs. If the fingertips of your O-ring don't separate very much, that question isn't the issue, because it's strong; it's not giving you an entry. If the fingertips separate a great ways, you've more than likely identified a real issue behind your health condition.

When you're first getting used to energy testing, it may take some practice to become comfortable with the arm test or the O-ring method. A good way to see if you're on the right path is to test your name. Say, "My name is," and state your name. The arm test or O-ring should be strong because that statement is true. Then try it again with a name that isn't yours. The test should be weak. Keep experimenting with this until you get accurate results. Then apply it to your health issue.

If, after you get the hang of energy testing, you ask all three questions and don't get an entry for your issue, try changing the direction of your test. For example, if you were testing for migraines, maybe the truth is that only 60 percent of what you experience are migraines and the other 40 percent are regular headaches. You can change the way you ask the question to something like, "Is this an issue or issues?" instead of "Is this migraine-type head pain an issue?" The word "issue" encompasses all possibilities, and you'll get an entry that way.

Even if you get an entry on the first or second question, ask all three of them anyway. You may find multiple entries. For example, migraines could really be an issue for you, and thinking about them could also trigger them as an issue. You want to cover all your bases.

Know. As soon as your fingers respond to your scan of the issue, you enter the last phase of ASK: know. You make no assumptions about what the result of your scan will be, and you allow that result to come to you. You're comfortable not creating an answer, because you know that the answer is within the question itself. At this point, you are in a state of neutrality, observing the result without feeling any attachment to it.

When you do gain an entry to your issue and your fingers separate, your neutrality is the open door that allows harmonization to take place. You literally harmonize the issue as soon as it registers, simply by identifying it and being neutral to it.

Harmonization does not mean that you are covering up your symptoms. By harmonizing the energy like this, you are actually going back to the time and space where the issue first occurred and inverting it. You are hitting an energetic reset button, and it's as if the issue never took place at all. In other words, you don't just feel better; you *are* better.

Once you've found an entry through ASK and harmonized the energy, you should feel an improvement right away. Take a moment to compare that feeling to the way you felt before. Then test the same question again, using the same process of ASK. Most of the time, you will feel stronger. If the test still gives you an entry, don't worry about it. Just perform the harmonization a few more times, until the weakness is gone. Eventually, you will harmonize yourself to your full, optimal potential.

Now, when you're testing like this, remember: energy goes both ways.

That means you're thinking about your migraines, and your migraines are also thinking about you. You may want to get rid of your migraines, and you may support that energetically. But when you test the energy, you may find that the migraines themselves don't support letting you go. However, whether the resistance is coming from you or the migraine, harmonizing the energy will improve the issue.

Always listen to the message the energy is sending you when you test, no matter where it's coming from. Don't just put your will out there. Be aware, and recognize what's coming back at you.

Want It, Need It, Deserve It

Using your GPS successfully can be attributed to your intention to shift your world simply by virtue of these four things: wanting to, needing to, deserving to, and finally being neutral to accepting the shift.

Wanting, needing, and deserving are really representatives of three different frequencies within us. Your want is your conscious mind, your need is your subconscious mind, and your sense of deserving is your soul. Your soul deserves a better outcome; it deserves to fulfill its karmic duty.

Once we harmonize these three frequencies using Guided Personal Source, we gain a greater sense of knowingness. The final piece of the puzzle is accepting that awareness, which comes through neutrality. Neutrality allows us to open our arms and say, "Yes, I'm comfortable with this. I'm okay with receiving the good things that are coming my way."

All of this is contained within you. Energetically speaking, your GPS is really independence. As long as you want it, need it, deserve it, and accept it, you might never need to depend on outside people or circumstances to move forward.

ASK Your GPS

Your GPS is all-inclusive of everything that you are. It contains all the probabilities and possibilities of what is creating your symptoms and how to shift conditions back into balance. Everything is self-encoded, self-sufficient, and self-intelligent. All you have to do is ASK.

That said, harmonizing energy is not a one-time deal. Energy is always in motion, and for your health to stay at its optimal potential, you need to keep up with the flow of energy. The next chapter will give you the tools you need to maintain energetic balance.

Chapter Five:

MAINTAIN ENERGETIC BALANCE AND NAVIGATE THE MORPHIC FIELD

Don't Go Back to Texas

I had a client named David who was diagnosed with terminal lung cancer. Traditional medicine had given up on him. "You have thirty days to live," his doctors said. "Get your affairs in order."

And he did. He told his family the news, and they began to arrange his funeral and everything down in Texas. David lived in Los Angeles at the time, but he planned to return to Texas to spend his last days with his family.

Before he left, however, he came to see me. I connected with his energy field and was able to harmonize his issue.

That was on a Friday. The following Thursday, he walked into my office waving an MRI in the air. "It's clear!" he announced. The tennis-ball-sized mass on his lung had completely disappeared.

"Great," I said, testing his energy again. "Your energy feels good. You can head home and return to your normal activities."

"Oh, no," David told me, "I'm going to move back to my hometown in Texas. All my family is there waiting for me. The doctors said this might be a remission, so I want to take the opportunity to be with them for however much time I have left."

As soon as he spoke those words, I felt the hair on the back of my neck stand up. A surge of energy went through me, and the news wasn't good. "Look," I told David, "do what you really need to do. But I test that if you do go back to Texas, you will have a relapse and you will not pull through."

Everyone in Texas was ready to bury him, I explained. They had it all planned out: the burial arrangements, the service, everything—all specifically timed to happen in thirty days. If he stayed in California, energetically speaking he'd be fine. But if he returned to Texas, his family's beliefs and expectations would very likely collapse into him and reverse his positive outcome.

"What?" David said. "No, that would never happen. They're my family. They don't want me to die. I'll show them that I'm better, and they'll be happy."

So David went back to Texas. And thirty days later, I got a call. He was back in the hospital on an oxygen machine, right about to cross over.

In the end, it wasn't cancer that killed David. He succumbed to the heartache and depression of his family's expectations.

Balance and the Morphic Field

Everybody is different, and everybody is changing—day by day and moment by moment. Maintaining energetic balance is like breathing: you don't just breathe once and say, "Okay, that's all I need." Breathing is a way of life, and balancing energy is the same way. We don't exist in a void. We live in a flow of energy that is always moving and interacting with us. That's why it's not enough to harmonize an issue once and forget about it.

To maintain energetic balance, you need to learn to use your Guided Personal Source to navigate the morphic field.

The morphic field was first identified by renegade British biologist Rupert Sheldrake in the twentieth century. It is an energetic field of influence created by the conditions around you. For example, you may have experienced the phenomenon of contagious yawning. You're in a room with several people, and one of them yawns. Before long, several other people are yawning, whether or not they actually saw the original yawn. That energetic influence is considered quantum entanglement at work.

We can be influenced by anything in any dimension of the universe, but the morphic field tends to be the one that we deal with most when it comes to maintaining energetic balance. That's because the morphic field is how we connect with everything and especially everybody in our lives. Your family members, friends, coworkers, and anything else in your environment combine to create your morphic field. And that morphic field has the ability to trigger your health issue by throwing you out of energetic balance.

The morphic field is not always a bad thing. If you go to a concert, the excitement of everyone being pumped up might affect you in a positive way. On the other hand, if you're going to Texas and your family is expecting you to die when you get there, the influence of the morphic field isn't a good thing anymore.

When it comes to maintaining energetic balance, the goal is not to change the morphic field itself. The goal is to have neutrality about where and where *not* to go so that we can decide where and where not to tap into it. This chapter will teach you about triggers and show you how to maintain harmony by navigating the morphic field.

The Truth about Triggers

The morphic field affects you through triggers.

A trigger can be anyone or anything. People, places, seasons, events, the weather—even thoughts can be triggers. Just thinking about a problem has the potential to trigger the actual issue, as you learned in the last chapter.

Some triggers are smaller than others. The case of David's family preparing for his death is an example of a very powerful trigger. However, at the end of the day, a trigger is a trigger, regardless of its size. It exists as energy, and it will affect you if you allow it to.

Triggers occur at multiple levels. Your symptoms may be triggered by one thing today and something else tomorrow.

For example, you may have triggers that affect you only at certain times of the year. Maybe every autumn at work, your boss tells you, "This is what our goals are." You're thinking, *Oh man, how am I going to do all this?* And it triggers your migraine. But ten months later, after you've already pulled most of those goals off, if your boss says, "Let's review our goals," you don't have a reaction to it. You know you're safe, so it doesn't bother you. Same topic of goals, but different circumstances.

Or let's say you've been eating a certain food all your life without any problem. Then someone comes along and tells you, "Don't you know that this food is carcinogenic?" Suddenly, you're worried about it, and that triggers you. You never had a health problem with the food before the trigger. After the trigger, you start to notice a difference, and you may even start to develop cancer. This is universal consciousness at work.

Things can be altered by the energy of a thought. This is called the observer effect. Nothing really affects you until you internalize it as an observer. At that point, it becomes a trigger, and you've got a problem on your hands.

Regardless of what your triggers are or where they come from, however, the process for dealing with them is the same. You just need to know how to navigate the morphic field.

How to Navigate the Morphic Field

To navigate the morphic field, you want to attain a state of optimal neutrality. I refer to this state as "naturally, neutrally normal." You are fully aware of everything you're seeing, but you're also neutral to those observations. This point of balance is like the equal sign between two halves of an equation.

For instance, let's come back to the migraine example. If you're dealing with migraines, then on one side of the equal sign you have the causes of your migraines, and on the other side you have migraines themselves. You harmonize the equation, and the migraines go away. But then you interact with the morphic field, and your mother says, "What? Your migraines can't be gone just like that. You've had them for thirty years."

If you're not neutral to that trigger, it adds information to the equation again—and you have to resolve it. But if you're neutral, then you're living on the equal sign itself. Nothing can be added to the equation, because you're not there to receive it. You're protected, because you're in a state of neutral energetic balance. Someone can say, "You should still have migraines," and your energetic response in awareness is, "I'm not going to go there, so don't bother me."

Here are some practical exercises for navigating the morphic field.

Test with Consistency

Because it's possible to trigger the same issue on different levels, for different reasons, one of the best ways to navigate the morphic field is to test your energy with consistency.

This doesn't mean you want to check it every day at exactly 9:00 a.m. On the contrary, by doing it that way, you're purposefully bringing your health issue to mind when you don't need to. Remember, even thinking about an issue can trigger it.

Instead, you want to test your energy every time you start to feel that you could use a tune-up.

For most people, that feeling of needing a tune-up kicks in when the harmonization of the issue drops below 65 percent of its optimal energetic correction. In other words, if you made your migraines 100 percent better using your GPS, you will still feel fine for a while even after triggers from the morphic field start to take a toll on you. As long as that harmonization holds at 90, 80, or even 70 percent of what you did originally, you probably won't notice any migraines.

But when you drop below the 65 percent mark, you start to notice the issue again. (To test your exact percentage, you can use an O-ring: say "10 percent," "20 percent," "30 percent," and so on up the list. When the O-ring stops giving you an entry, you've hit the mark.) That's when you want to start testing, ASKing for answers with your GPS just like you did the first time around, using the same process I explained in chapter 4.

The difference is that now, even though the process looks the same on the surface, you're actually going deeper.

Every time you do maintenance testing on your issue, you achieve a deeper level of correction as a result of your expanded awareness. You eliminate more and more triggers, leaving you with less and less to work on. And that means you experience your issue less frequently.

You can also test your issue more comprehensively, rather than testing for one specific thing, to make your energetic state as strong as possible. For instance, say you get migraines every time you visit your family for the holidays. You harmonized yourself for it last year, but now you have to go back for another round. Even though you're going to be seeing the same family members as last time, they're not the same energy that they were before.

You can actually test the future energy of that event before you ever get there, and the best way to do it is to use a phrase along the lines of "anything and everything regarding this issue." You could go through one by one and list every possible migraine trigger you can think of—your brother, your sister, your mother, the food, the cat, and the rest—but if you do it that way, you risk leaving something out. When you test for anything and everything regarding your issue, past, present, and future, that encompasses the whole myriad of things you'll encounter in the morphic field.

You don't have to know exactly which triggers you're harmonizing. The energy knows what the problem is, and it will make sure that you are strong and neutral—especially when you test with consistency.

"Invert Neutral Now" (INN)

You can also reapply the energy work you've already done on your issue—as well as address any new triggers that might show up after the harmonization has been done—using a GPS tool I call "invert neutral now," or INN.

INN is an integral part of your GPS, and the words "invert neutral now" are designed to restore and transform. "Invert" means that the energy of the issue never happened in the first place. "Neutral" is the act of letting go and having no attachment to the outcome so that your desired result can come to you. "Now" puts you in the moment, where everything exists and is available to you.

Let's say you harmonized yourself to 100 percent of your infinite potential using ASK. You felt great for a few days, but little by little triggers in the morphic field caused that good feeling to weaken. You're thinking, *Hey, I already dealt with this. I just want to reapply the harmonizations I already did.*

You can reapply the work you did before, using INN, like this:

1. Close your eyes and bring to your awareness the thought of what you want to change or restore. Take a deep breath in and let it out.

2. Open your eyes, bringing the palm of your hand up in front of you and placing the thought of what you want to transform and change on your palm.

3. Bring your upturned palm to your heart chakra (chest area), maintaining the thought of what you want to change as you do so.

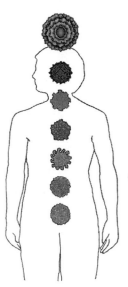

Crown Chakra
Color-Violet: Spiritual connection, understanding, knowing, bliss, oneness.

Third Eye Charka
Color-Indigo: clairvoyance, psychic abilities, imagination.

Throat Chakra
Color-Blue: speech self expression.

Heart Chakra
Color-Green: love, balance, compassion.

Solar Plexus Chakra
Color-Yellow: mental functioning, power, control, freedom to be oneself.

Sacral Chakra
Color-Orange: emotion, sexual energy, creativity.

Root Chakra
Color-Red: Kundalini energy, instinct, survival, security.

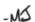

4. Say to yourself (out loud or in your head), "Invert neutral now." Take a deep breath in and out and let go of the thought of what you wanted to change or restore as you exhale.

5. Allow your hand to fall away from your chest, and feel and see the transformation as done.

Another way to use this exercise is to state, "Application of the harmonization that pertains to me now," in place of "invert neutral now." This simply reaffirms the energy work you have already done in a more specific way.

Performing INN is like refreshing a computer page. Just like that, you're good as new.

In Balance with All Things

Once you understand how to navigate the morphic field, you are in control of your own outcomes again. A doctor can tell you, "You've got thirty days to live," and you can say to yourself, "I don't see an expiration date stamped on my toes, sir." Your own energy, in the form of Guided Personal Source, gives you your last word, not the people or things in your environment. And that's the way it should be.

As I said earlier, even though we focus on the morphic field, you can be energetically affected by many other fields in the universe. The good news is that the state of neutrality can protect you from all of them. As long as your intent is to maintain neutrality, triggers will not be a disruptive influence in your health or in your life.

The deeper you go with testing and maintaining your energetic balance, the more harmonious and neutral your life becomes. You can think of yourself as a dusty house. The more you navigate the morphic field with neutrality, the more sweeping and cleaning you do, brushing away the dirt and clutter and returning to your natural state of total perfected essence.

In the next chapter, I'll walk you through some of the most common health issues and give you a behind-the-scenes look at what they often have in common, energetically.

Chapter Six:

COMMON HEALTH ISSUES: AN ENERGETIC VIEW

Olivia's "Tissue Issue"

When you test the energy to the source of an issue, it's almost never caused by what the doctors think it is.

Olivia was nine years old when her parents brought her in to see me. She had been diagnosed with Ewing sarcoma, a form of bone cancer, and the doctors said that she had less than a month to live. When she walked into my office, she was pale and emaciated, doubled over in pain.

I didn't assume anything judging by the look of the child alone. I tested her energy field using ASK. The energy field said that Olivia was out of balance because she'd had a parasitic twin—a brother in utero who never made it out of the womb. His cells were in her body, causing this cancer. They just needed to be harmonized.

So that was what I did. I facilitated the harmonization of those cancer cells. I consider cancer cells to be a form of life, not death—living cells that are opportunistic in nature—but they didn't belong here. Incidentally, doctors in the medical profession have come up with chemotherapy agents that seem to mimic what I do energetically, in the form of chimeric antigen receptor—or CAR—T-cell therapy. The difference is that they use chemical agents to target and kill cancer cells, while I energetically harmonize and invert the life force of the cells so that the individual in question is no longer a host.

Immediately after I facilitated the harmonization, Olivia's appearance changed. Her color came back. She stopped holding her tummy and sat up straight, the pain gone. She was surprised, but her mother was taken aback. "That's impossible," she said. "All the doctors said there was nothing we could do."

But Olivia felt fine. They'd flown in from out of state, and when they got back to their hotel, she jumped in the pool and started swimming.

After Olivia went back home, her doctors couldn't figure out what was going on. "Your daughter's lab results indicate that she should not be doing this well . . . but she's clearly improved," they marveled.

That's because energy has its own logic. Olivia didn't care about lab results. Olivia cared about living, breathing, and playing. And she went right on with her life.

Behind the Scenes of Health

Everyone is different, and every health issue is different. You don't manifest exactly the same migraine as the person next to you, and your migraine isn't caused by exactly the same thing that triggers the other person's migraine, either. The knowledge of precisely what's going on in your case is something that only your Guided Personal Source knows.

At the same time, patterns of energy do occur and can be identified among some major health issues in general.

For example, something that many health issues have in common is a weak thyroid. Medical science is beginning to catch on to this, but I test far more connections between health and thyroid malfunction than the medical establishment is currently aware of. Health issues can also come from energy fields off the body, and they can be triggered by literally anything at all.

If you limit your awareness of what causes health symptoms to what you read in traditional medicine books alone, you're unlikely to get to the bottom of what's really causing your issue. But if you begin to think about those symptoms in a broader way, you expand your awareness and become better prepared to receive the real answers when you ask for them.

This chapter will broaden the way you think about health conditions by sharing with you some energetic commonalities that go beyond the limits of traditional medicine. Keep in mind that all of these patterns are relevant to actual issues, and that sometimes the issue can be created simply by thinking about it.

Some of the most common health conditions I address in my practice include issues such as addictions, AIDS, Alzheimer's and dementia, asthma, autism, autoimmune disorders, cancer, cerebral palsy, colds and bronchial infections, diabetes, heart disease (including blood pressure and cholesterol), hypertension, infertility, Lyme disease and Morgellons, multiple sclerosis, nervous disorders, obesity, renal failure, vertigo, and vision issues. Let's take a very brief look at each of these in turn.

Addictions

With addictions, a person may be energetically weak or strong to whatever the addiction is. The addiction can also go both ways. For example, if someone is an alcoholic, I test the energy to see whether the person is holding on to the alcohol or the alcohol is holding on to the person.

People can also take on addictions as a way of covering up other issues that are going on with them, such as depression, schizophrenia, or bipolar disorder. Energetically, it's important to get to the bottom of the mental issue driving the addiction. Stress, anxiety, tension, multiple personalities, and seasonal affective disorder (SAD) also scan energetically under "addictions." OCD patterns can sometimes cause an individual to hold on to an addiction, and I likewise test for those when I'm working on addiction issues with my clients.

AIDS

AIDS often tests back to the left side of the body on the spleen, which is one of the largest organs in the lymphatic system. I normally energetically track the condition back to when it first occurred and then correct it, harmonizing the field so that it never happened.

AIDS is an autoimmune disorder, and I usually recommend supplements such as natural immune boosters and high doses of vitamin C to support the energy work that's been done.

Alzheimer's and Dementia

Alzheimer's and dementia energetically tend to be associated with a certain receptor on the back of the brain. I test that receptor, and it tells me that the brain and nervous system are short circuiting. A short circuit means the brain isn't getting the message.

I often track the source of the problem back to heavy metal exposure on the left receptor side of the body. That tends to indicate the involvement of dental work or other forms of environmental toxins that the person may have had in the past.

With Alzheimer's and dementia, there's usually scarring in the brain as well. Most of the time, it comes from things such as bad diet, the environment, and chemicals such as smoke that irritate the linings of the blood vessels. My Alzheimer's and dementia clients do well with brain rejuvenator support or electrolytes to support their energetic harmonization.

Asthma

Asthma is the perfect example of a condition caused by triggers. Usually, the triggers are either emotional or environmental. For example, a teacher might be heading to a class where she really doesn't want to see a number of particular students, because they're always causing trouble. The thought of those troublemakers upsets her, and she starts hyperventilating. This is a classic asthma scenario.

Autism

Energetically, I find that not all autism is caused by vaccines, but some vaccines can cause autism or autism-like conditions.

Parents often bring their autistic children in to see me, and if I test that autism is really an issue, then the next thing I test is when the issue began. About 80 to 90 percent of the time, the condition started two weeks or so after birth. As soon as a baby is born and washed, the first thing most hospitals do is vaccinate that child with a hepatitis B shot. The energy shows a two-week incubation period before the nervous system begins to deteriorate and the baby begins to have neurological symptoms. With the other 10 or 20 percent of autism cases, the issue began in utero.

Once I identify when the autism occurred, I harmonize the field by clearing that time and space, which resets the pattern of the energy field to the person's brain. Combined with some nutrition, I find that these cases do very well.

Autoimmune

Autoimmune disorders are conditions where the body fights itself. The most common disorder is Hashimoto thyroiditis, which can end up leading to scleroderma, lupus, and everything else.

When I test the energy, I usually find that the person has been exposed to an allergen or poison that triggers the body's self-resistance. Vaccines are a prime example of this. They trigger the body to fight against otherwise normal things, such as peanut oil, which is used in most vaccines as an excipient, causing the body to recognize it as a foreign substance. Once the field is harmonized, the individual can stop having a negative reaction to peanuts.

Cancer

I refer to cancer as a "tissue issue." Most people think of cancer as death, but it's actually life. Energetically, you can have cancerous elements in your body and still be perfectly healthy, as long as the energy flow to the cancer is "turned off," or harmonized. The left side of the body tends to metastasize more readily than the right side. Once you identify the cancerous field, it's usually open to change, shift, or dissolve.

In many cases, cancer comes from a twin complex that took place in utero. Just as with Olivia's unborn brother, we sometimes hold on to parts of our siblings' bodies. When those superfluous body parts are "turned on," cancer can develop in any number of forms. I turn it off by harmonizing the field, and the person gets better.

Cerebral Palsy and Muscle Weakness

With cerebral palsy and muscle weakness, the brain isn't getting the message to the muscles, and the muscles can't respond well. The person can't control his or her gait, movements, or speech. Rarely, the muscles themselves can carry issues, such as a spindle fiber with a protein deficiency.

The block in communication between the brain and muscles is usually the result of an obstruction in the flow of impulse between the muscles and the nerves. This is similar to what we find in multiple sclerosis, where the sclerosis prevents the nerve impulse from moving to the muscle from the nerve. Harmonization corrects the problem.

Colds and Bronchial Infections

Colds and bronchial infections are signaled by receptors on the lungs. From there, I test to see whether the infection is bacterial, viral, or fungal. Fungal infections are the worst, followed by viral infections, and bacterial infections are the least serious.

The infection isn't always limited to being just bacterial, viral, or fungal. You can clear up a fungal infection only to have it become a viral infection, and when that clears up you can still have a bacterial infection. Whatever the case, you just reset the immune system, and the issue will be corrected.

Diabetes

Type I diabetes is a condition that usually has its beginning in utero and can sometimes have its beginnings in other life forms from previous lives. Type II diabetes is often the result of diet and lifestyle.

Energetically, I always test the pancreas and the specific cells within it: alpha, beta, delta, and the islets of Langerhans. Whichever of those cells gives me a reading is the culprit of the diabetes, and I invert the energy to harmonize it.

Cactus, cinnamon, and especially bitter melon are the best supplements I've found for supporting balanced blood sugar.

Heart Disease, Blood Pressure, and Cholesterol

With heart disease, blood pressure, and cholesterol, the energy usually tracks back to a circulatory issue that is affected by the thyroid. I also see a pattern with blood vessels collapsing in the coronary arteries. They're like water hoses: when water (or in this case, blood) flows through them, they expand, but when the flow stops, they collapse. Much of the time, these issues can be hormonal, especially when they are thyroid related.

Hypertension

I usually get a reading on hypertension by testing whether there is a reflex to it on the bicep muscle of the arm. When hypertension is an issue, I often track it to either the heart or hormones—and those two are related. The person may have low hormone levels of testosterone, progesterone, estrogen, or even adrenaline. Because of the lack of hormone support, the heart has to pump faster to keep up. I normally harmonize the field and support the thyroid with iodine so that it will produce the correct hormones and the heart won't have to overwork.

Infertility

Infertility usually tests as being hormone based. Most of the time, the woman has estrogen dominance, and there's a lack of progesterone. After I invert the energy field, I often recommend progesterone cream as a supplement. I avoid progesterone suppositories, which are usually rejected by both the body and the baby.

Liver Disease

The most common thing I see with liver disease is toxin congestion. These toxins can come from an individual's environment, diet, dental work, or even cuts on the skin. I usually harmonize the field and recommend a detox program along with electrolytes and other supplements specific to the individual.

Lyme Disease and Morgellons

The root of Lyme disease is almost always specific to a deer tick, and it comes with an energetic pattern of chronic fatigue syndrome. If the fatigue syndrome is very strong, I test to see if it's Morgellons, which is a broader autoimmune condition that can be related to other pathogens in the system. In both cases, the spleen usually shows up as being weak when I test the energy.

These conditions are often contracted one or two years before any symptoms show up. I track the energy back to the time that it occurred and invert it, and the symptoms go away. I also recommend a supplement for autoimmune support, such as colostrum, to support the energy work.

Multiple Sclerosis

Multiple sclerosis is caused by calcium deposits in the ventricles of the brain. The energetic harmonization dissolves and clears the calcification so that the brain comes back online, and there's a greater flow of spinal fluid. After I reset the pattern, the area improves. I usually recommend zeolite combined with minerals to rejuvenate the brain.

Nervous Disorders

Nervous disorders include conditions such as Parkinson's disease and Lou Gehrig's disease (ALS). With nervous tics and disorders, a commonality I find is that the pineal gland isn't getting the message across the blood-brain barrier. The proper neurotransmitter in the brain isn't getting where it needs to go, and the result is that the nerves misfire in a loop that never ends, like a broken record. I reset the receptors in the pineal gland and support the harmonization with electrolytes, and the condition improves.

Obesity

Obesity often isn't truly an issue. It can be an emotional protection that a person has developed over time, safeguarding him- or herself against other threats. These individuals feel safer that way, so they hold on to the weight. This is very common. When obesity is in fact an issue, it's usually related to a weak thyroid.

Renal Failure

Environment is one of the biggest factors in renal failure. Exposure to toxins, heavy metals, high proteins, and chemicals in the body often turn out to be the cause of failed kidneys. Your kidneys are like filters, straining proteins and other nutrients from the blood. When the filter clogs, you develop problems. Excess protein in the urine can be a cause of swelling and hypertension.

Cysts or kidney stones can block the function of the kidneys, and kidney stones are usually the result of calcium imbalance.

Vertigo

Vertigo and dizziness are usually triggered by something in the environment that causes an allergy in the ear—almost always the left one. I often track the vertigo to the client's left ovary or testicle. Most of the time, it's related to a testosterone deficiency and is easily corrected with harmonization and supplements.

Vision Issues

Vision issues are often connected with brain issues. We think we see with our eyes, but we really see with the optic nerve of our brains. If the brain is calcified or has heavy metal poisoning, it causes vision problems.

Another common vision complaint is cataracts. You don't necessarily get cataracts as a result of wear and tear on your eyes, such as prolonged exposure to car headlights over the years. Instead, they can be caused by tight muscles from strained vision. Once the muscles relax, the cataracts go away. "Floaters" in the eyes are often caused by calcium and mineral deposits.

As with everything else, harmonizing the energy improves any kind of eye issue you might have.

Targeted Energy Testing

You do not need to be able to test for the exact time, place, or energetic field of a condition to harmonize it. Again, energy is self-intelligent. When you work with it using the tools you learned in the previous chapters, it will find the right time, place, and energetic field for you, and you will experience positive results.

That said, some individuals are curious to know what the exact cause of their condition is. These causes can range from karmic issues to emotional issues to experiences from previous lives, and the list goes on and on. It's possible to identify these references, or triggers, and knowing the exact triggers of your condition can help your healing to go deeper.

I teach students how to identify triggers in my courses. If you would like to learn more about this, you can visit www. garciainnergetics.net.

Health and Beyond

You can see that there's more to your health than you may have thought. Full health is not simply the absence of disease. It encompasses the physical, mental, and spiritual. And health isn't the only area where you can use your Guided Personal Source to tap into your infinite potential to transform your outcomes.

Literally everything in your life can be tested on the same energy grid on which you test your health condition. Moreover, everything can be harmonized using the very same tools you use to improve your health. In chapter 7, I'll show you how you can apply what you've learned to the other areas of your life.

Chapter Seven:

Beyond Your Health

Wish for a Well

Anita was a student of mine from Northern California, and she needed to dig a well.

She hired a company to do the drilling; for a large sum of money, they gave her three chances to find the water vein. Obviously, Anita didn't want to go into the venture blindfolded if she could help it. So she hired someone with a divining rod to help her locate the water, and she used what she'd learned from my classes to search for it herself.

After two tries, the drilling rig came up dry.

"All right," Anita said to the drillers, "hold on. Before you continue with the third spot, I need to consult with someone to find out where that should be."

Then Anita came down to see me, bringing a map of the property with her. Without showing me where the first two drills had been done, she asked me where I thought she should drill the third one.

I tested the energy and touched a corresponding spot on the map. "Right here is where I get the best reading," I told her. "How far away is that from where they dug before?" Anita looked at me. "That's about a foot away from the last hole," she said.

When she told me that, I had to double check myself. It was only a foot, I thought. What's the difference? I tested it again, and then again. Each time, the result came back the same. "Yes, that's the spot," I said. "The energy is telling me that that's the most optimal place to dig."

Even though it sounded crazy, Anita trusted me, and she trusted the energy work. She went back to her drilling team. When she told them that she wanted to drill the third hole only a foot away from where she'd dug the last one, they thought it sounded crazy, too. "You know, most people go at least ten or fifteen feet away," they advised. "You have a lot of land to work with."

"No, no, dig right here," Anita insisted. She'd been close to the target with her original energy test, and we had both agreed on the spot, so at least she wouldn't feel guilty if she missed. "I've already spent the money. Let's do this."

Sure enough, they hit water. Not just a little water, either: Anita found such a huge gusher that she had enough water to provide for her entire town. In the end, hitting the well had been like hitting a vein when you draw blood: you can be close, but if you don't get it at just the right angle, you're not going to have enough pressure, and it's not going to work.

After the fact, Anita admitted to me, "Yeah, I was in the vicinity, and they were also in the vicinity with their divining rod. But it didn't give me the results that you and I got together."

Expand Your GPS

Everything is energy, and energy is everything. Up until now, you've been tapping into your GPS with the specific lens of health in mind. But while answers to your health issue are powerful, they're really just a drop in the bucket of what your Guided Personal Source has to offer you.

Literally anything in your life can be tested and harmonized with energy using the same energetic tools you use to improve your health. Your GPS is more than just a manual to diagnose your physical symptoms. It is your energetic signature. You can use it to test the energy of absolutely everything you can imagine—and then some.

For example, a lot of clients come to me for energetic readings about prospective business ventures. These are high-powered people, and they want to make sure they're investing their money wisely. I'll test the energy and tell them, "Hey, this is a bad deal. But we can correct it energetically."

You can do more with energy than just see what outcomes will be. You can harmonize the field to create the outcome you wish for.

In this chapter, I'll show you how you can apply the energetic tools you've learned to different areas of your life, including money, finance, relationships, career, occupation, and future and life purpose. I'll also explain how you can help others with the same harmonizations you use to correct yourself.

Common Life Supports

Almost every non-health issue that my clients bring to me scans energetically under a number of categories. These categories include money, finance, relationships, career, occupation, and future and life purpose. We all deal with each of these in our daily lives, with relationships and future coming up as the most common triggers.

Here are some examples of each of these life supports.

Money

I define money specifically as physical cash—what you have in your purse or wallet. It's actual, concrete currency. Dollars and coins. You can hold it in your hands.

Some people are weak to holding or having money. For example, in some cases, their grandparents told them that money is dirty. This is especially true of grandmothers. They'll say things like, "Don't touch that, it's dirty! Don't put it in your mouth!" And that idea rubs off on the individual in question, who will carry credit cards or checks around just so that he or she doesn't have to handle money itself.

When you work on harmonizing this, you're really correcting yourself to be okay with the energy imprint of money. Beyond the physical money itself, you might also have an issue at the particular time that it was printed, or with the symbols printed on it. For instance, you might be weak to money printed on September 11, 2001, because it carries the energy frequency of the tragedy that hit the World Trade Center. Or you might have lived a previous life during the Civil War, and as a result you have an aversion to bills printed with Ulysses S. Grant's image.

I held a workshop once where one of the students had a resistance to money. When we got to the money and finance part of the class, she spoke up and said, "Oh, I've always had issues with money."

So I had her come to the front of the room, and I worked on her energetically. Her GPS told me that she was weak to twenty- and ten-dollar bills, and she also had a particular weakness to coins. So I corrected her and sent her back to her seat.

When she went to sit down, coins started falling out of the sleeves of her sweater.

They were everywhere. Everyone in the room turned to look at her in bewilderment, speechless. She had the same expression on her face as she looked back at us. "I don't remember having any coins in there," she admitted. The money had come in from another dimension or universe.

One thing was clear: she didn't have an issue with money anymore.

Finance

Finance covers the scope of money that goes beyond the physical currency itself. Credit cards, investing, net worth, and bank statements all scan under the finance category, energetically. The profitability of investments and the rise and fall of financial markets can be tested using energy work.

Refinancing for a loan is a common event that falls under finance. You need to demonstrate that you have a certain amount of funds on paper before the loan goes through. I myself had an interesting experience with this.

When I first applied for a refinance loan, my real estate agent gave me a call. "We can get the loan," he told me, "but we have to show the bank that you have a certain amount of funds in your account by five o'clock today."

There wasn't any doubt in my mind that I would have enough funds to pay the monthly mortgage. Still, I didn't have the needed funds in my account right then. Worse, I was at work and couldn't leave. "Okay," I told my agent, "just hang on a minute. Let me try something."

Energetically, I tested the account I had at my bank. My testing revealed that the funds were present in several other parallel universes. I connected with one of these universes and energetically brought the required amount—which was a frequency of energy, just like anything else—into the now moment, dropping it into my account. The funds were not a new apparition. Rather, they had always been there.

My agent was still on the phone, looking at my account, and he didn't miss a beat. "Oh, I don't know what you did, but it's there," he said lightly. "I think we got it. I'll call you back." We hung up.

Sure enough, he called me back later and said, "We got the loan."

"Great," I said, and I just went on with my life. I didn't even think about the money in my account. It had done what I needed it to do, and the task was taken care of. Then, at the end of the month, I received my statement and found to my surprise that the money was still there.

My wife and I were amazed. We had no idea that it would do that. But in the end, that wasn't the point. We thanked Source for providing what we needed to carry out the work.

Relationships

Relationships aren't limited to people alone. Remember, energy goes both ways, and you are always in an energetic relationship with everything in the field: you to money and money to you, you to your health issue and your health issue to you. This is why relationships are often the biggest thing in the energetic field to work on, and they encompass a lot of emotion.

Now, that said, relationships between people are a big factor in the clients I see. Someone will come in and say, "I have an issue with my spouse. He doesn't listen to me." I test the energy, and often it's a communication issue. But not always.

One client of mine, Linda, came to see me because she was concerned about her teenage daughter, Mindy. Her daughter was about to start college, and Linda was worried that Mindy wasn't quite ready. This was putting some strain on their relationship.

"Why do you feel that Mindy isn't quite ready for college?" I asked her.

"Well, when I was her age, and I was going through a similar process of looking for the right college, I didn't feel ready to be on my own," Linda admitted. "I felt pressured, and I had no real direction of where to go."

I tested the energy and found that Linda was projecting her past experience onto Mindy, which wasn't serving either of them. So I harmonized the energy between mother and daughter, inverting it to release Linda's attachment—a form of quantum entanglement.

On her next visit, Linda had good news.

"Mindy found a college," she said with a smile. Her daughter was happy there and was doing very well. Linda herself was calm and at ease, having let go of what she considered "mother-daughter" issues.

The strain between them was gone, and the relationship was optimal again.

In relationships, it is important to test for any ancestral patterns or issues that we might have between one another. This is especially valid in family dynamics, but applying a harmonization is also a good idea with relationships you may have with work colleagues, business contacts, or anyone else in your life.

We live in a world of many different ethnic and religious backgrounds. As a result of this, we don't always agree or get along, but we need to work together to make the world a better place. Harmonizing the energy field with regard to relationships is a significant step forward in this direction.

Career

Your career is your professional title and overall field of work. You can use energy work to direct you to the right career or advance the career you're already in. For example, you can harmonize your business to help it reach its maximum potential, or guide your decision as to which career to start in the first place.

One client of mine had a son, Matthew, who was looking for some direction with regard to his future career. Matthew was about to graduate high school, and he was thinking of going into the health care profession. Specifically, he was interested in working on injured athletes as an athletic trainer or physical therapist.

"I'm not sure about it, though," he admitted. "I'm worried that I won't be successful in health care."

I tested Matthew's energy and found that health care was a strong option for him. Encouraged, he went to school and did very well, completing his studies as a physical therapist. Soon afterward, however, he switched to the chiropractic profession.

"Why did you switch?" I asked when I saw him, surprised.

"Because of the energy work that I saw and experienced with you during our sessions," he told me. I'm a chiropractor in addition to an energy facilitator. "I want to do more of what you do."

To this day, Matthew is one of my intern facilitators in my energy classes, and he applies what he himself has learned in those classes to his busy chiropractic practice.

Occupation

The relationship of occupation to career is similar to the relationship between money and finance. While career is the big picture of your profession, your occupation encompasses the specific, concrete activities you do on a daily basis. For example, if you're an engineer, you might have no problem with that career field in general, but you could really dislike one specific task that's required of you at work. You don't need to change careers. You just need to harmonize yourself to that particular task.

For example, one of my clients runs a business in which she sells her products to vendors. She had no problem with the business itself. But she was getting tangled up in the ground-level transactions of doing business.

So I harmonized the field for her. "Look," I said, "you've got to reverse your approach to this. These people that you just had a meeting with aren't your only option. Others are going to be calling you up, and they're going to want your product. You don't have to worry about it. They need you more than you need them."

As soon as I spoke the words, an email alert sounded on her phone. She checked the message. "Oh my god, a new person just came in. She really wants my stuff!"

I just nodded and said, "You see how fast it works?" She's been having greater success with her occupation ever since.

Future and Life Purpose

We all have a tendency to worry, "What's ahead for me?" A very common subset of that is life purpose. "What is the meaning of life for me—now and in the future?" A lot of people are afraid of success and being in the spotlight. Or they think, "I don't deserve this. It can't be this easy." All of that relates to future and life purpose.

You can harmonize yourself and correct the field for whatever is going to happen. You don't need to imagine what's going to happen, because the field already knows. The harmonization will make sure that your future reality is optimized as the perfect time and space. Some people are weak to the terminology of "future" or "life purpose." Sometimes people have no problem with the future, but the future has a problem with them. Remember, energy goes both ways.

One of my clients had a retail business that helped a lot of people, but she felt like something was missing. She wanted to be more present and to see the value of what she was contributing. She wanted to understand the purpose of her existence.

I harmonized her and recommended that she just allow things to happen as opposed to proactively trying to make things fall into place. She took the advice, and her whole life turned around—her business, her finances, her outlook on the future, everything.

Most of all, she identified her life purpose. It was her, herself. She became her own person, and growing into that awareness gave her an enormous sense of happiness and empowerment.

Treat yourself for the future while you're in the moment. After the harmonization, you'll feel better, and good things will come to you just as they're meant to. Live in the "now" energy. As Eckhart Tolle says, "If you are truly conscious, your life grows quickly stronger."

Help Others with Energy

The work you do with energy isn't limited to what you can do for yourself alone. You can use these same tools to help others as well. You don't even have to be in the same room. You can work on people—and anything else—remotely.

The reason that's possible is that everything is energy, and energy transcends time and space. You can tap into any field using the same techniques you use on yourself. Working on others isn't more difficult than working on yourself. In fact, a lot of the time it's actually even easier, because you're more neutral to the result you're trying to achieve.

DISTANCE ENERGY HEALING

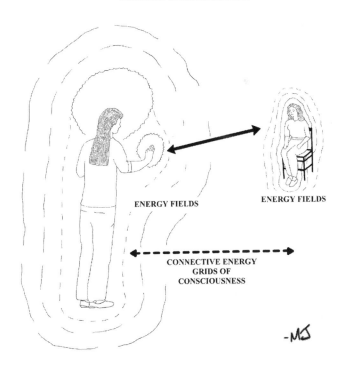

ENERGY FIELDS   ENERGY FIELDS

CONNECTIVE ENERGY
GRIDS OF
CONSCIOUSNESS

-MS

For example, I've helped people in different states and countries with their health issues without ever leaving California, where I live. I've harmonized the weather when it would have ruined an important national outdoor sporting event.

On one occasion, a woman called me about her dog that had just been diagnosed with lymphoma, and the vet said that the animal probably wouldn't make it. I tested the energy remotely, found that the dog had gotten the infection from stepping on some metal six weeks before, and inverted the field. Right away, the dog was fine again.

Working on others remotely is that easy.

Now, when it comes to facilitating energy for others, some people ask, "Wait, aren't you interfering with the free will of those people if you work on them energetically? Aren't you interfering with their karmic debt?"

The answer is no. You're not interfering with anyone's free will through energy work, because ultimately the person you're working on has free will to accept your harmonization or not. If I pray for someone, that person doesn't have to accept the prayer.

As for karmic debt, energy work doesn't interfere with that, either. The individual still gets to experience all of the necessary events. The difference is just that, after the harmonization, you're experiencing it as a fender bender rather than a head-on collision. The essence of the event itself is still intact.

Helping others with energy work is something I go into in greater depth in my classes. To learn more, you can visit www.garciainnergetics.net.

Your Energetic World

Everything exists as potential energy, meaning that it has the potential to effect any outcome. All we have to do is allow it to transform our intention into reality. That is our Guided Personal Source: it guides us by allowing us to test what is available to be harmonized.

Your GPS will take you anywhere you want to go in your personalized energetic world. If your career has to do with finance, you can use energy to test finances. If you're in real estate, you can use it to test the housing markets and harmonize the energy there.

You have a fully equipped toolbox, and you're free to allow whatever results you want. Your intuition will guide your creativity from there. When you truly tap into it, you will improve not just your health, but your existence and your whole awareness of the universe.

The last stop on your energetic journey is also the first one: Source. I'll show you how your GPS keeps you constantly connected to "home base" in the next chapter.

Chapter Eight:

YOU AND SOURCE ARE ONE

"You'll Never Walk Again"

Robert was on the ground, mangled and bleeding after a horrific motocross accident, when he somehow managed to call me. He was in his mid-fifties, and he was one of my students. When I tested the energy, I saw the damage he'd taken: broken legs, snapped spine, and a ruptured midsection, among other things. I was amazed that he was still alive.

Both Robert and I immediately started connecting with his energetic field—I was doing my part remotely—while emergency personnel got him into an ambulance and took him to the hospital. When he got there, they said that he should have bled to death on the course, and it was clear that the work we'd done energetically had saved him. But he wasn't out of the woods yet.

"You'll be lucky if you live," the doctors told Robert. "And even if you do, you'll probably never walk again." He was paralyzed.

Robert stayed in the hospital for a month, induced in and

out of a coma by the medical personnel so that he wouldn't bleed to death. All the while, I continued to remotely connect with him energetically. When they released him, he was in a full body cast. He couldn't bend his body at all.

Nobody believed that Robert would be able to get out of bed and move—except Robert. "I'm not hanging around just to wither away," he said. "I'm going for this."

He insisted on making an in-person appointment to see me soon thereafter. My office is on the third floor, and the elevator was broken that day. When I drove back to the building after my afternoon break, I saw Robert in his full-body cast at the foot of the stairs. *Oh man, I have to hurry up and go help him,* I thought. But by the time I parked and got out, he was gone. He actually beat me by taking the stairs to my office on the third floor. "How did you do that?" I asked when I saw him.

"Oh, you know, I just did the energy work," Robert said, "and I went for it."

Robert came in to see me every other month for six months, and he worked on himself energetically between visits. He maintained a positive outlook on life. By the time those six months were up, he had significantly improved and was moving as well as he had before the injury.

In the end, Robert didn't just walk again. He returned to doing most of the other activities he'd enjoyed before the accident as well. And he did it by leveraging the healing power of energy.

He did it by tapping into the part of him that was Source.

You and Source Are One

As I've said before, the mind is a terrible thing to use, unless you control it. Up to this point in your life, you may have been buying into the emotional illusions around and within you, such as "I'm worried" and "Why me?" These are side effects of letting the mind run wild through a mirage of problems and uncertainty.

The truth is that problems and uncertainty aren't real. Our minds create them. When you put the tools you've learned in these chapters to work in your life, your Guided Personal Source takes over, and the illusions of problems can no longer fool you. In other words, your mind doesn't run you anymore; you run your mind. And you do that by developing your intuition.

You do it by allowing yourself to be one with Source.

Source is where intuition comes from. It is energy itself. And remember: energy doesn't always follow human logic. But it does always know what's truly in your best interest at any given moment.

In the emotional chaos of life, we forget that we are more than our physical body. We forget our perfected essence, and we feel disconnected from our divinity. But disconnection is the illusion. You can't be disconnected from what you are. And what you are, at your core, is Source.

This chapter will show you how to deepen your intuition and give you the resources to continue learning about energy work, if that is the path that feels right to you.

Develop Your Intuition

Developing and deepening your intuition is like anything else: the more you use it, the more you'll have available to you.

The more you are in the field of energy—testing situations on a daily basis—the easier it becomes to facilitate the energy itself. Your field becomes more harmonious, and so does your daily life. In other words, practice makes perfect. But I don't mean that in the usual way.

When most people think of practicing to get better at something, they think of it like a chore. They feel like they have to set up rules and regimens and force themselves to go through certain motions every day. But the truth is, the more you think you have to go to work on something, the only thing you're going to do is create more work to do—and that's limiting, not to mention unenjoyable.

You will never find a question with a fixed answer when you work with energy, because energy is not static. It is living, evolving, and infinite—and it is personal to the individual. That's why regimentation doesn't work. That's why it can't be boxed into a system, and why it can raise and mold consciousness.

Practicing energy work isn't about regimens. It's about learning to be in and of the field so naturally that it becomes second nature, allowing the energy to give you exactly what you need to have in order to accomplish the end result. The more you allow things to come to you, the more effortless it becomes. And the greater your awareness of energy, the more the energy becomes aware of you. "Oh, Hector is looking for this," it says. "Let's provide it for him. Let's help him out."

In a way, facilitating energy feels like the concept of "let go and let God." But the truth is, it's even more than that. As I mentioned in chapter 4, you can have all the potential energy in the universe at your disposal, but without your intention to give it direction, it's not going to give you what you want. No one else can do that for you. Neither can this book.

Outside elements can only trigger you to want to take the journey. You are the one who actually walks the path. You are truly unique, with your own authentic signature, soul purpose, and contribution to make to the world.

Use the framework and exercises you've learned in these chapters to get you moving in the direction you want to go, but don't think of them as the be-all and end-all of working with energy. Instead, use them to springboard you into a new way of living, a new way of being.

The more you awaken and develop your intuition, the more you'll be able to neutralize the emotions that go along with the mirage of disconnection from Source, whether you're dealing with health or any other life issue.

Receive What You Deserve

One big obstacle that gets in the way of many people achieving their full potential as a facilitator of energy is the question of deserving the results they get. They feel like this whole method of working with energy is too easy. They think they should have to work hard at it before they can earn such incredible results.

Here's the problem with that outlook: if you feel like you have to earn something, then what you're really saying is that you don't already have it.

You are Source, and Source is you. You are a hologram of an all-encompassing field of energy. The sense that you need to earn your good results in order to deserve them is really your ego getting in the way, driving a separating wedge between you and your perfected essence that does not actually exist. It's part of the mirage. Every time you do that, you're setting yourself up for limitation and failure.

With energy, all things are possible, especially when you are in harmony with the universe. Remember that it is easier to do what is right for the universe first. When you align yourself with that intention, you will receive anything and everything that you deserve.

Infinite Learning

Now that you've read and internalized the information in this book, you've crossed a threshold. You have the option to use the already powerful tools you've learned and stop there, or you can choose to go even deeper into what energy has to offer you.

If you decide to go deeper into energy work, you don't have to make that journey alone.

The tools you've learned in this book are powerful, fundamental. They can make an enormous difference in your life. Even so, it's possible to go much deeper with them. Many people enjoy the support and various perspectives of honing their energetic facilitation skills in a group setting.

The classes I host give individuals of all experience levels and from all walks of life the opportunity to grow their knowledge, pick up new tools, practice on one another, ask questions, and experience the power of the work firsthand. Energy work at a distance and learning to identify specific triggers from any of the twenty-two fields of energy are also covered in the class.

Teleclasses are another avenue for continued education and learning. Many people find these accessible, because they can call in from anywhere in the world without having to be present in person. Garcia Innergetics hosts teleclasses once a month. You can learn more about our workshops and teleclasses at the back of this book.

Many of the people who learn the Garcia Innergetics method say that their whole lives have changed. "I get up in the morning, ask what's new for the day, and harmonize my field. My business is a lot better, my relationships are better, my health is fantastic. It's amazing," they tell me.

The potential for the lives they're now living was in them all along. And now, they know how to access it.

Thank You for Being Source

At the end of every session I do with my clients, I reinforce the work that was done with one last exercise. I say to the individuals I work with, "I want you to tap into your original perfected essence."

As soon as they do that, the transformation is obvious. Their bodies become lighter and relaxed. I feel their souls evolve as they tap into their spiritual body, which happens to be Source. Source is perfect, and so are they. They become integrated with that perfection.

When I ask them how they feel afterward, they tell me, "I feel comfortable with myself. I feel whole. I feel complete."

You are that perfection. And now, you are in a position to recognize it. You have access to the guidance of personal Source—the self-intelligent knowingness that you came here with, and that you'll take with you when you leave. You are tapping into that intelligence as opposed to going outside yourself in search of it, returning to your original essence.

Energy goes both ways. You were searching for something that would help you with your health issue when you found this book. But the book also found you. You are ready to tap into your intuition. You are ready to access the universal awareness that will allow you to tap into any field of energy and say, "I am confident enough to make the right decisions in my life."

The moment you do that, you are doing more than helping yourself. You are improving the quality of the universe itself. You are in Source, of Source, and you are Source. That is the ultimate gift, to you, from you, and for you.

Thank you for being Source.

TRANSFORMATION BEYOND THE BOOK

Now that you have experienced *Guiding Personal Source*, if you would like to deepen your awareness by learning more about your GPS, Garcia Innergetics, and other subjects covered in this book, you can do so by visiting www.GarciaInnergetics.net or by calling our office at (858) 450-9221.

You can also attend one of Dr. Garcia's live workshops. These classes are a simple-to-understand and easy-to-use hands-on experience using a combination of live lecturing, demonstrations, and guided practice. Students receive a manual which mirrors the Power Point presentation given during the lecture, with added space for taking notes. You can expect to have fun, laugh, and gain an expanding knowledge about energy work. A great benefit of the workshop is that when Dr. Garcia is working on and demonstrating with one student, the whole class receives the benefits of his energy work, as well. These workshops are open to anyone and there is no prior experience necessary to begin your journey to a better, more harmonious life. Additionally, Dr. Garcia gives live tele-classes, which dive deeper into the subjects discussed in his workshops.

If you are ready to begin your journey of transformation, visit our website and sign up for a class today.

www.GarciaInnergetics.net
(858) 450-9221

40628150R00069

Made in the USA
San Bernardino, CA
24 October 2016